# trash the trophies

## HOW TO WIN WITHOUT LOSING YOUR SOUL

# CHASTA HAMILTON

# HOUNDSTOOTH
## PRESS

TRASH THE TROPHIES

*How to Win Without Losing Your Soul*

ISBN   978-1-5445-1428-4  *Hardcover*

       978-1-5445-1427-7  *Paperback*

       978-1-5445-1426-0  *Ebook*

trash the trophies

*For the people of Stage Door Dance Productions: you all have truly taught me how to "Be More At Stage Door."*

# CONTENTS

# FOREWORD

I first met Chasta in 2007, when she was the coach of my dance team during my junior year of high school. We moved around a lot when I was a child, and dance was the one thing that remained my constant. I had a lot of dance teachers, and I can say, without hesitation, that Chasta is the one with whom I connected the most. She was young and enthusiastic, which of course, made her way more relatable to me than my older and more "traditional" dance teachers, but beyond that, she had a spark. At the time, I could not pinpoint it, but there was something about her that made me feel I could accomplish whatever I set my mind to.

As I came to know her, I started to recognize that she was much more than a phenomenal dance educator; she was an incredible human who had a mission to truly leave the world a better place. It didn't take me long to learn that she could (and would) accomplish literally anything she wanted. As our dance team coach, she would always give us crazy choreography for the skill level of the team (she chose not to cut anyone who auditioned because she wholeheartedly believed in everyone), followed by an inspirational pep talk. One of these pep talks ended with, "Don't make excuses; make it happen." While I think that this was something she came up with on the spot, it is something that has stuck with me and is what I think best represents who she is.

Our dance team ended the same year it started, but I'm lucky our friendship didn't. I so vividly remember the day Chasta called me to tell me she had signed the lease for her own studio—a goal that she had set her mind to and made happen with no excuses. She was still young, I was entering college out of state, and I remember her talking about the studio with such passion to create a happy and magical place of inclusive dance education. I saw the studio being built, was there for some of the very first classes, and although I was out of state in undergrad for the first few seasons, it was my second home in the summer and on breaks. I would always look forward to teaching camps, guest classes, and of course, choreographing for the competition team.

See, I grew up at studios that competed; it was almost like competitive dance studios were equivalent to higher dance training. In other words, if you wanted to dance at a high level, you competed. If you didn't, you "just danced recreationally." If the studio was going to be such a happy and magical place that pushed kids to their fullest potential, why wouldn't we offer competitive teams?

After undergrad, I moved back to Raleigh as the Assistant Director of Stage Door Dance Productions and remained there as I worked my way through graduate school. As part of this job, one of my main responsibilities was to coordinate our competition team. While this started out as something fun and exciting, with parents who were grateful for additional opportunities and more intensive training, it quickly turned into the complete opposite. Shows about the competitive dance industry were being aired on national TV, and the industry started quickly shifting to an environment driven by profits, popularity, trophies, and made-up recognitions for the sake of giving every child an award. With this shift, there were more competitions, more awards, more nationals, more conventions. Every competition became completely subjective and lacked consistency across the scoring and the judging—a concept that was very hard for parents to understand. As teachers, we were on the front end of communication, and it was not easy to explain to a parent why a child may have received the "rising star award," a platinum adjudication, and second overall at one competition and solely a High Gold adjudication at the next. It became exhausting for us, our staff, and honestly—the children. It was easy for kids to post things on social media, see awards won by other studios, follow other dancers on various social media platforms, and utilize those social media platforms to develop a self-image of what kind of dancer they *should* be based off the one(s) with the most followers.

Exhausted, burned out, and dreading competition season, Chasta approached me one day with the idea to cut our competition team and switch to a noncompetitive studio. I will be the first to admit that I was apprehensive. After all, 90 percent of my time was devoted to building relationships with our competitive dancers and parents. How would that impact the studio? How many people would leave? If competing was how dancers received more intensive training, what would happen to our clients if we said we were taking this component away?

Then, one thing happened that made me realize this wasn't such a bad idea after all: burned popcorn.

As part of being a larger, competitive studio, we spent an incredible amount of time planning summer intensives for our students. While we opened them to any dancer wishing to participate, they were mainly attended by our competitive dancers and often coincided with some sort of competition choreography for the upcoming season. We would use these intensives to expose our dancers to a variety of styles and teachers with the idea that it would help them develop well-rounded training. We started with local talent and guest teachers, but eventually, parents would attend conventions, see big names teaching, and request that those teachers guest-teach at our intensives. We also realized that more dancers would attend if we reallocated our budget to bring in these "big names."

With insane teaching rates came hotel rooms and food stipends, so we often only brought in a few of these artists—but it kept the dancers happy, which kept the parents happy. One summer, we brought in a guest artist who was featured on multiple TV shows, taught at conventions we attended, and was well received by our dancers and parents. This guest artist flew in one evening and was scheduled to fly out the next day after a day of teaching. Since we always provided transportation to and from the studio, we made sure any guest artists who needed overnight accommodations stayed at the same hotel. This night, one of Chasta's friends was guest-teaching as well and had arranged to carpool with this other person to get to the studio the next morning for classes.

It was that morning that Chasta received a call from her friend that our "star" guest artist's room was completely engulfed in lingering marijuana smoke. Chasta called me to ask what our best course of action would be. Fortunately, this person did not seem under the influence at the studio.

Our first course of action was to immediately place another

studio staff member in the room during this guest artist's class to ensure the instruction was quality. The guest artist was leaving immediately after classes, so they were not going to be returning to the hotel. We had the keys to the room, as we generally handled checkout. We hopped in the car and headed over to check things out. After all, if it was as bad as it was reported, we didn't know if authorities would be involved (remember: this was in the early years of the studio when marijuana was still criminalized in North Carolina), or if at the very least, we would be charged for smoking in a nonsmoking hotel.

Well, we get there and notice the McDonald's trash from the previous night and the unmistakable smell. We did the only thing two stumped problem solvers know how to do and jumped on Google. We were quickly informed of the one thing readily known to cover up the smell of marijuana: burned popcorn. Who knew? We sure didn't, but it makes sense.

So, while our dancers and staff were learning from this well-established and respected artist, feeling as if they were receiving the best training out there because of this person's resume, Chasta and I were in the recently vacated hotel room burning popcorn to cover up the smell of stale marijuana to avoid receiving a smoking charge on top of all of the other fees we had paid to bring this person to the studio. This was the turning point for me.

It wasn't the hundreds of parent emails I received expressing concerns over artistic choices we made that season, awards ceremonies that lasted until well past 1:00 a.m., eighteen- to twenty-hour days at competitions/conventions without seeing the light of day, or sleepless nights wondering if what we were doing was good enough. It was the burned popcorn that made me realize we didn't need the competitive industry to be successful, and that our dancers would be better off if we channeled our time and energy into providing both excellent dance education and skills that our dancers could use to thrive beyond the studio.

It's been a few years since we transitioned out of the competitive industry, and I can honestly say that walking away was one of the best decisions that we could have made. I eventually went on to receive my master's in counseling, PreK-12th Grade Educator's License, and accreditation from the National Board of Certified Counselors. I worked as an elementary school counselor and served as a director for a local nonprofit, but I somehow manage to always find my way back to the studio. I truly believe that this is because it is now finally that happy, magical place that Chasta dreamed of so many years ago.

Our dancers are happy, our parents are happy, our staff is happy. We are giving our students skills that they need to be successful in life and preparing them for the world outside of high school. Children as young as eight are coming into the studio with ideas on how to support local community organizations, people (children and adults) are kind to one another, and there isn't jealousy sparked by meaningless competition adjudications or resentment fueled by the outcome of awards ceremonies. Our dancers are hosting shows/events and raising funds that are truly making a difference in the world. Children are starting to see that you don't need an award to be rewarded—rewards come when you become your best self and positively impact the lives of others.

So, am I anti-competition now? No, I'm not. In fact, from my professional experience working with children, I believe that healthy competition is necessary for developing basic life skills, such as sportsmanship, perseverance, and goal setting. Yet, the dance competition industry's environment is not healthy. Over-rewarding children with participation trophies, made-up awards, and defining success based off of the subjective opinions of a few select judges is ultimately doing a huge disservice to our future generation.

As educators, we have the privilege of working with and shaping children every day. So why not take advantage of this opportunity and teach all children how to set goals that will truly better themselves and make a difference in the community? It's time for us to stand together and use our time, energy, and resources to teach the importance of setting meaningful goals and being good people.

It's time that we model how to use our skills, passions, and talents inside and outside the studio to positively impact the lives of others. It's time that we trash the trophies. After all, a diamond or crystal award has never determined one person's ability to succeed, and one's self-worth is defined by way more than the number of followers they have on social media.

Oh, and if you can relate to anything that I've said or if you truly feel that this is what you need to do to improve your studio culture, your quality of life, and the dance education your students are receiving, then I leave you with words from one of the smartest and most credible women I know: "Don't make excuses; make it happen!" You CAN do this, and I guarantee you will feel so much better once you do.

—SARA THAMES, MA, NCC

# INTRODUCTION

The bass was booming on a Saturday night around 11:00 p.m. as Taylor Swift's "Trouble (Goat Remix)" blared on the numerous video screens that surrounded the stage. I was working my seventeenth or eighteenth hour of the "weekend" at a dance competition with students from my studio. My glasses were on because I had pink eye in both eyes. Exhausted and unhealthy, I was a walking representation of physical and emotional burnout. As a naturally enthusiastic person, I felt more like a shell of myself, a walking robot moving through the motions, prepared to address concerns and facilitate negativity. With tears in my eyes and a knot in my throat, I chose to sit off to the side to quietly reflect on the mess in front of me.

As expected, one of my dancers was called to the stage as a mega-winner of the weekend. I sat in my seat cringing because I knew I was going to be invited on stage to share in the victory. When it happened, I walked up, prepared to fulfill my obligation. I stood on the stage of the Durham Performing Arts Center, a 2,712-seat venue, feeling hollow and defeated. Lights were flashing and songs were blaring. Sensory overload is an understatement.

"Hug your dancer!" the emcee enthusiastically said as though this moment should represent everything I ever wanted for my entire life.

I exchanged gestures, but it was meaningless.

Just like the entire competitive dance industry.

If you've spent forty-hour weekends at regional events or your ten-day summer family vacations at Nationals, you've probably had similar fleeting thoughts. When we convene for these events, we lose our weekday identities of business owner, husband/wife, lawyer, chef, room parent, doctor, and honor-roll student and instead transform into Dance Mom, Dance Dad, Dance Competitor, and Number-One Dance Teacher. We sacrifice healthy meals, sleep, and our sanity to keep the ruse going. The aggressive desire to win is all-consuming.

Even if a parent suggests they're simply participating "for the fun of it," it is probably through a forced, fake smile that is slapped on as a response to societal standards versus genuinely authentic feelings.

When we are positioned in our "Dance Competition Roles,"

- We root for some children to win and some children to lose.
- We experience every range of emotions imaginable.
- We feel super confused about consistency in scoring.
- We make friends, lose friends, and discover our real friends.

And we wonder, why are we doing it?

I lived this full range of emotions alongside my clients in nearly every city across North Carolina, up and down the East Coast, and in randomly scattered locations like New Orleans and Anaheim.

Our happiest moments were always tied to the joy of performance without awards. One time, one of our little guys was tearing up the Cha-Cha Slide on stage prior to an awards ceremony. Our dance families were in fits of joyful tears and jubilant laughter over this display of pure, organic performance. It represented everything dance can and should be!

A few minutes later, an awards ceremony started and,

because this child didn't achieve a top-ranking trophy, the mood immediately darkened with accusations of being "robbed." It completely erased the joy and community we had experienced. In a quick second, we went from a collective ensemble to a hungry pack of wolves. And the catalyst of the response: a trophy.

What's the price of this type of behavior and environment?

- An immense amount of time.
- An exceptional amount of money.
- Emotional and physical exhaustion.
- The false sense of validation of approval from an industry that has no regulation and hypocritical standards.

As invoices containing alarming amounts of entry fees due crossed my desk, I knew I would never pay this amount of money for my child to participate in something so superficial. If you can't fully support something, how do you sell it? I longed for the program to be something I could celebrate and wholeheartedly support.

There had to be an alternative option for heightened dance education that was truer to my purpose. Success and victory had to be achievable in a more meaningful way.

That feeling is the motivator that prompted me to make a major change.

Late one night, under a blanket of stars and a cloak of humidity, I dragged trash bag after trash bag to a discreet dumpster. I wanted to be somewhere else far, far away, but my mind was focused on precariously guarding the careful disposal of each bag. I feared the strange objects would pierce the sides and be visible to the public. It'd be fitting; the past few years had certainly been thorny. Though part of me was longing for the simplicity of days gone by or some (really, any) sense of normalcy, I knew it was time to move forward and embrace a new era.

I was trashing the trophies and leaving the competitive dance industry behind.

My decision wasn't easy. It was two years in the making as I quietly watched the competitive dance industry wreak havoc on my dance studio business and my legacy. I faced pushback from clients and staff and wrestled with my inner conflict as well.

The trophies didn't represent success or victory. It was quite the opposite. They represented hurt, stress, toxicity, and anxiety. They marked a period in my career where my dream was tainted, my legacy compromised, and my future unknown.

Self-care wasn't on my radar. Books about being a badass didn't feel encouraging, and day after day, I felt like I was drowning in a sea of negativity. There were secrets, betrayals, and enough drama to fill an entire soap opera series.

As the intensity continued to escalate, there was less listening and more directional confrontation: "You should do this! You should do that!" The noise was deafening, and I reached a breaking point that forced me to listen to my voice.

When I made the decision to trash the trophies and leave the competitive dance industry, I made it out of the need for survival, but I knew that if I went all in, I could do something that hadn't been done. I could PIVOT, I could DISRUPT, I could REMODEL not only the dance industry, but the entire perspective of the children's extracurricular market.

With a heightened focus on social marketing, return on investment, community and culture, and all-in impact, the world was craving connection, and I craved change. I was being pushed to the edge, but in this horrible challenge, there was the greatest opportunity of my professional career.

We all know the gut feeling, the instinct, that's so easy to ignore but sickening to acknowledge. It can be professional, personal, or societal. Take my story and know that while my experience may not be the same as yours, we ALL have the power to shift the narrative when our lives and our dreams feel derailed. Action is what matters the most!

The twelve chapters of this book are centered around action-affiliated steps that will allow you to take control of your story in a successful and victorious way that is free of meaningless insignia.

1. Start a Fire. If you could do one thing for the rest of your life, what would it be? Why? How do you identify and eliminate distractions that contradict your passion and purpose?
2. Ride the Roller Coaster. Is the ride worth it, or are you bending your standards to conform?
3. Stay Alert. When something feels off, inventory it and activate a plan.
4. Make the Moves. Use your voice for things that matter, even when it's inconvenient.
5. Prepare for the Storm. Emotionally prepare for the transition, and strategically navigate and communicate the change.
6. Own Your Narrative. Build the buy-in through identifying (and owning) the meaning and messaging behind everything you do.
7. Level Up. Use your rebranding to correct missteps and exceed expectations.
8. Change the Game. Are you a complainer or a game changer?

9. Be Bold. Know the traits of bold leaders, and rock them.
10. Show Your Strength. Follow these tactics for tenacity and the importance of forward motion.
11. Pave Your Path. Navigate the noise with your words and actions, paving a path that represents you.
12. Let's Launch It! It's go time!

While the examples in this book are specific to our experience exiting the competitive dance industry and creating a new program and model that are aligned with our purpose and mission, the themes are universally applicable to any person's professional and personal fulfillment. What holds you back? What weighs you down? What is keeping you from being the best, most fulfilled version of yourself?

I am a forward-moving person. I do not like to look back, because it slows down progress. This book was hard to write. I had to revisit a lot of unpleasant memories and mistakes I made as a leader. With every passing year, I gain more clarity in the vision and realize the power in the choice I made. While your industry or circumstance may not be the same as mine, your power to cultivate change is real.

You see, *Trash the Trophies* doesn't solely symbolize the need to strip away labels that are counterintuitive to our personal and professional success. It's a calling to alleviate any distraction or relationship that interferes with our path and purpose. It's about awareness, readiness, and complete commitment to elevating your field of opportunity, whatever that may be.

*"If you don't like the road you're walking, start paving another one."*

—DOLLY PARTON

I grew up in the land of Dolly Parton. A regular season pass holder to Dollywood and a child of Lisa Frank and the Delia's catalog, I believed in rainbows, butterflies, Polly Pockets, and dreams.

The hills that raised me are officially labeled Mohawk, Tennessee. It's a small land where imagination makes anything possible. In those hills, I wanted to learn as much as I could about everything. I read books, loved school, and independently led my own research projects on topics that fascinated me. I craved knowledge. More than knowledge, I craved the opportunity to get out and see the world.

In 2003, the opportunity to get out presented itself in the form of a full, $150,000 Park Scholar academic scholarship to North Carolina State University in Raleigh, North Carolina. While my college peers were getting in on the ground floor at Google, I was struggling to find my identity and self-worth. Was being an artist a professionally respectable career choice? Society doesn't really promote that as an option, so I went down the smart, basic path of pursuing a career in law.

Throughout college, I wrestled with the rattlesnake of imposter syndrome, and after being completely unfulfilled in an internship with the North Carolina Attorney General, I abandoned that path and discovered my entrepreneurial spirit. I had an insatiable desire to prove myself, and I decided to do that within the dance industry instead of the legal field.

I am grateful I had the fortitude to pursue the career path that would set my heart and mind on fire. I've always been a Type A hustler. Success has always been the only option. Malcolm Gladwell would attribute this to my categorization as an "eminent orphan," claiming that "the death of a mother or father is a spur, a propellant that sends them catapulting into life. Because they are on their own, they are forced to persist, to invent, to chart their own way..."[1]

I didn't lose a mother or a father. I lost both. When I was two years old, my father died heroically in a trucking accident. When I was nine years old, my mother died heroically after an intense battle with breast cancer. My aunt and granny heroically raised me and graciously supported every non-conventional whim and passion I decided to explore and follow.

---

1    Malcolm Gladwell, *Outliers: The Story of Success* (New York: Back Bay Books, 2011).

I never spent a considerable amount of time sharing this piece of my history with many people because, even at an early age, I felt like labels can misrepresent a myriad of preconceived notions. I never wanted people to assume anything I accomplished was for any reason other than exceptionally hard work. I remember walking out of high school one day and a kid flippantly saying, "Oh, you only got that scholarship because your parents are dead." Absurd. I talk about it all now because, with experience, you gain the understanding that owning your past is key to claiming your future. There's power in acknowledging the pain, but it certainly doesn't define your existence.

My story led me to where I am today.

Listen up, because:

- Your story is what makes you capable of surviving.
- Your story is what gives you the ability to ignite change.
- I'm learning that it is empowering, and I bet you will, too.

As an only child living this wildly abnormal childhood, I spent a lot of time fostering my creativity. I talked to myself from sunup to sundown and played with my Barbies until I was entirely too old. I had imaginary productions, dance studios, businesses, and classrooms. Whenever the opportunity presented itself, I would coax anyone in my vicinity to be in my productions, begging them either to participate or to watch the latest vision in my mind.

I was always slightly interested in being cool, but never interested enough to actually be cool. I hit trends a few months past their time and never quite made it to the "cool crowd" in the social hierarchy of middle school, high school, college, and, well, life. I never wanted to watch R-rated movies without parental permission, and I didn't drink alcohol until I was twenty-two. I was the epitome of a rule follower. A unifier versus divider, I've always attempted to avoid conflict and criticism and achieve happiness—*attempted* being the key word.

When I opened the first location of my dance studio, I was opening the doors to my heart and the art that had so graciously kept me on a focused, intentional track as I navigated my childhood trauma. The performing arts heal, and I wanted as many people as possible to share in their organic power of therapy. I'm an eternal optimist, so it seemed like a no-brainer in my mind.

In execution, it was slightly more complicated. When business meets art, it becomes like setting choreography. How do you balance passion and profit? I was always creatively minded, but I did not always have the business acumen. It takes time to find a rhythm and culture. Who will you be? What will you represent? How do you balance innovation versus what's already happening and/or what's already been done? When others push their influence upon you, how will you stay strong and true to your vision? In the process, there were missteps.

The missteps we experienced involving the competitive dance industry shook us to our core.

*Chapter 1*

# START A FIRE

What could you do all day every day for the rest of your life? For me, the answer is easy. I've always loved the performing arts. Give me a show, a song, a big dance number, and I am one happy girl. I've always known what I loved, but I didn't always know why I loved it.

I opened Stage Door Dance Productions in Raleigh, North Carolina, in June 2009—right smack dab in the middle of the housing crisis and recession. My ego was youthfully strong, and nothing was going to get in my way. While "bubbles were bursting," I was fearless and ready to take on the world. I knew the dance world better than anything else. I was committed to offering the best of everything I had experienced as a student, as a teacher, within other dance studios and businesses, and of course, in my imagination.

In our first year as a studio, I believed in all the good in the world. I thought everyone was equally passionate, good-hearted, and excited about the art of dance. We were going to kumbaya and kickball change together in perfect harmony.

I was eager to jump in and take the world by storm. I received my certification from Carolina Dance Masters/Dance Masters of America, a nonprofit, educational, competitive circuit that requires members to test via exam for inclusion.

Once our programming was up and running, I was eager to submit students for competitive events in their fall cycle. It seemed fun, and it seemed like the thing to do to increase our reputation as a strong, new dance training facility.

I was in it to win it and was excited to receive all the trophies—the bigger, the better!

Looking back, the naive, slightly reckless, youthful excitement is so evident. I was impatiently ready to achieve victory. I don't regret it, because the intentions were pure, but there was so much to learn about people, the process, and the overarching purpose.

The parent of one of the participants of this "jump in/take on the world initiative" was very upset when her child did not qualify to advance to the next round at the first competitive event we ever attended. It was a "Title Competition" where the top ten dancers from each division advanced. This child did not advance. (Side note: none of my students advanced.)

Instead of the dancer walking away from the event with a fired-up motivation to continue her growth and training goals, the family misplaced the blame on inappropriate placement in our dance classes. I had never experienced a reaction like this, so I was blindly entering this situation. We didn't always have opportunities like this growing up in eastern Tennessee, so I was excited to be a part of it all. In time, I knew we could work our way to the top, and I was ready to lead the way.

After the mother expressed immense frustration with my incapability to achieve results for her daughter, I responded in writing. Here is an excerpt from my response:

> "At our studio, we do not separate recreational and competitive dancers in their technique. Instead, we offer high-quality technique instruction to all our students...I must reiterate that at our studio, we are not all about winning. While the competitive event may have been disappointing, it should be viewed as an educational opportunity. We are not going to win everything..."

As a more seasoned business owner rereading the conversation, I recognize that my entire explanation was too long, unwarranted, and likely fell upon deaf ears. I strive to use my words more wisely now, but even in our earliest days, I knew that our studio and our success would not be built upon trophies or winning. I had conviction! I envisioned a synergistic educational component combined with a positive and motivating environment. It takes time and experience to identify and uphold your core values.

The situation with this parent rapidly turned into a classic "grass is greener" fiasco, and unfortunately, I did not have the confidence in branding and culture to articulately navigate and command the situation. The gist of the response was that the mother respectfully disagreed with my recommendations for placement. At the time, I was flabbergasted.

There were two pieces the parent shared in the exchange that weighed heavily on my heart.

My first (and, unfortunately, not last) encounter with the train-up mentality:

*"It is my belief that if you are surrounded with people with similar or greater skills, you are pushed to perform at a higher level. If, on the other hand, you are in a group of people with much less experience, it takes time to develop certain skills before more advanced techniques can be learned."*

My first (and, unfortunately, not last) encounter with the must-win mentality:

*"We certainly understand you can't win them all. However, it is difficult when you work hard, and the results are not what you hoped for or expected. Everyone loves to win."*

The parent closed the email correspondence with this quote:

"As simple as it sounds, we all must try to be the best person we can: by making the best choices, by making the most of the talents we've been given."

Yes! That's what I was trying to accomplish. So, where was the breakdown in communication? How did we so quickly go from being on the same team to being in opposition?

My initial reaction was to question what I was doing wrong. When I make a mistake, I want to own it and attempt to make it right. The child was in a group of similarly aged and skilled peers. She was working hard and being challenged. As an instructor, I was taking my role of challenging her very seriously and made sure the entire team was looped in on this student's goals.

Ultimately, this was a classic lesson in blame displacement. I didn't understand it at the time and would face it multiple times before I learned to recognize it in advance. The catalyst of this situation?

The competitive dance industry.

There's no book or class that prepares for situations like this (the closest one is *How to Win Friends and Influence People* by Dale Carnegie, which I read multiple times that year). Instead, I relied on the advice and perspective of experienced women I admire. I was leaning in before Sheryl Sandberg labeled it.

One of my mentors sent me the following nuggets of wisdom:

- Dialogues/debates do not often lead to resolutions
- Stay above the content that isn't directly applicable to your program. Emotional issues, family matters, and the like are things you cannot control.
- Be aware of bullies! They may try to force their philosophies on you (e.g., a love of winning), but you do not have to bend your ideologies to conform to their beliefs.
- Value your time and be purposeful with communications.
- Stick to your decisions.

This conflict continued in an escalation to our billing department. The family never officially submitted a withdrawal notice, and a confirmation of program departure was necessary. Isn't it interesting how the most difficult clients have the easiest time bending the rules and manipulating the expectations?

The response I received included the most personally painful words to date:

> "You would think that a smart business owner would try to keep and appreciate the few clients/dancers that you have. As opposed to running dancers and staff away. You have yet to prove yourself in the dance world to have this kind of attitude..."

Ouch. Exhausted, fatigued, and disappointed that I could not please this client, I closed out the exchange with a final round of communication. It probably wasn't heard, but it felt necessary.

You know how they say history repeats itself?

It does.

This was the first of many intense dialogues that stemmed from discontent surrounding the competitive dance sphere. How do you work to your fullest potential when your purpose and passion are constantly being questioned or attacked?

Students and employees cannot thrive with high levels of negative feedback, and business owners cannot be expected to thrive in a constantly negative environment, especially when the negativity is provoked by a third-party industry. How do you improve something that is completely out of your control?

Recently, I had a casual conversation with one of my best friends, Sara, a guidance counselor. She mentioned that a healthy ratio of positive criticism to constructive criticism, a ratio of 4:1, generates productivity. In the depths of our competitive experience, our ratio was majorly askew.

While the challenges often felt overwhelming, each one was an eventual invitation for the opportunity to reinvent and creatively discover a better way to build a business, create a brand, shift expectations, and fulfill purposeful legacy.

The enlightenment surrounding why I love the performing arts entered my life on a hot August night at Yum Yum Thai Restaurant in New York City. I was dining with my friend Mike—a friendship that blossomed (ironically) through the competitive dance industry. Three hours in, we talked about everything I had going on and where I could stand to "trim some fat" in my professional endeavors. He's an incredible leadership coach, and he wanted to workshop some exercises.

In going through the material, I realized the pieces of my professional life that spoke the most to me were the ones that involved empowering and inspiring others through the performing arts. Yes, I loved the performing arts, but I especially loved using them as a vehicle to empower and inspire others. That's what really sets my heart aflutter! When you know this information, a wave of clarity washes over you, and you want to act on the purpose-filled path as quickly as possible.

At that moment, I passively recognized that participating in dance competitions, as a judge and as a studio, may not be the best representation of my purpose. When something threatens to fizzle your flame, especially when your fire embodies passion, hard work, dreams, and livelihood, raise the red flag and hit the brakes.

Positioning, particularly from multiple angles, is power. Discovery and facts help us understand the full landscape of a situation. Education and experience lead us to informed decision-making. This is an industry I lived in through many different iterations. I've been a winner, a loser, an observer, an insider, and an outsider. In transforming from being all in to being all out, there's a lot of opportunity for thought and reflection about the good, the bad, and the ugly. All of it is necessary to keep your fire fueled and your passion active, alive, and aligned with your mission and your purpose.

*Chapter 2*

# RIDE THE ROLLER COASTER

I've always had a love/hate relationship with roller coasters. From a young age, I hated the idea of them and would cringe when spotting the looming, tall structures in the distance as we entered theme parks. From the Georgia Cyclone at Six Flags in 1994 to the California Screamin' at Disneyland in 2012, the sheer terror and excitement of the ride represented a thrilling, personal conquest. I'd drive myself crazy with anxiety waiting in line and getting into my seat, scream like a banshee during the ride, and feel victorious as ever once my feet hit the ground. I love the memories of laughing over my ridiculous faces in the souvenir pictures as you exited the ride. The mix of joy and terror was real!

In thinking about the competitive dance industry experience, the journey mirrors a long, drawn out roller coaster ride. I would always get on the ride because I'd rather be included in the action than be an observer from the outside. How often do we bend, sacrifice, or compromise our standards to fit the status quo? Society says roller coasters are fun and thrilling, so we ride them, even if it isn't really our thing. Society suggests dance competitions are a way to prove value and worth in your dance education business or dance training, and we go along with it, even if it isn't really our thing.

The competitive dance industry is this weird, gray space between performing arts, deregulated youth sports, and a propaganda-fueled megacorporation. The sparkling trophies and hazy messaging are a dreamy opportunity to participating students (and parents!), but the reality is the glitz and glamour come at a significant price, literally and figuratively.

A dancer's competitive routine roster at his/her studio may include solos, duos, trios, small groups, large groups, and "line/production" routines. The general fee structure for competition is based on the number of participants per dance. From our experience, entry fees are scaled, with solos being the most expensive, duos/trios falling in the midrange, and group routines being the most economical.

At The Dance Awards, a national competition experience,

the pricing is published as follows: $155 per three-minute solo, $80 per participant in a three-minute duet/trio, $65 per person in Group (4–9 participants), Line (10–15 participants), Extended Line (16–24 participants), and Production (25+ participants). Group and Line receive three minutes on stage, Extended Line receives four minutes on stage, and Production receives five minutes on stage.[2]

(Note: these figures are from an upper-tier Nationals experience. Pricing can vary within $20–$40 of each itemized entry fee, depending on the size and production value of the competitive event.)

For the business of dance competitions, solos are the least profitable. Why? If you have a group of sixty students performing together in a "Production" at $65 per head, the competition is bringing in $3,900 in revenue in a five-minute period. Cha-ching! Yet, solos are the most alluring for participants, so students and parents pay 100%+ more than the group routine cost to watch their child shine on stage (alone) for three minutes.

Let's pause for a second.

Before I continue, think about the last time you spent $155 on a 3-minute experience.

---

2    The Dance Awards, accessed April 24, 2020, http://thedanceawards.com/competition.

As a comparison, here are some other ways you can spend that amount of money to enhance your dance training:

- Two and a half hours of private dance or vocal lessons in Raleigh, NC
- Six ninety-minute group classes at Broadway Dance Center in New York City
- One Broadway show or national tour ticket (approximately two and a half hours of entertainment)

When a dancer competes, he/she must also purchase a costume to complement each routine. In the competitive dance industry, this may include custom-designed apparel featuring thousands of Swarovski AB Crystals.

Years ago, the most basic custom costume might cost in the range of $500 per design. The custom designs are not couture creations like you see pop stars wearing on tour; instead, it is a basic variation of a bra and panties with ornamental decoration applied. If you opt for a pedestrian costume or a catalog costume, the cost is likely going to be in the $50–$100 range.

To gain a scope of the level of participation, some competitions limit solos to four per participant. During the peak of our competitive dance tenure, some dancers would perform in thirty to fifty routines in a weekend. If you do the math, that's an alarming amount of money in entry fees.

Aside from entry fees, some events also offer an educational convention component, which basically means hundreds of dancers packed in hotel ballrooms with renowned (sometimes "celebrity") instructors sharing their knowledge. The convention component usually costs an additional $250–$300 per event.

It isn't hard to hit $1,000 per competitive weekend in entry and educational fees. In addition to those weekend costs, there's also the costs of traveling/lodging for the event, training, costumes, and any additional studio-incurred fees (music editing, instructor travel, etc.).

If a participant or his/her parent experiences addiction to the accolades, they may choose to travel city to city, hoping for a shot at the isolated bubble of competitive dance fame. It's an isolated bubble because the experience really doesn't duplicate any actual piece of the entertainment and performance industry except for the literal fact that it is a performance happening on a stage.

The rules pages for competitions are individually created and mimic legislative documents to address ethical issues such as studio-hopping, mixing ages to win, instructors performing with dancers, and the number of acrobatic skills that can be performed in any given routine. There's also an appropriateness clause, which everyone loves to publish and proceed to ignore, because, in the same vein as the entire industry's business model, there's an abundance of gray space, politicking, individual opinions, and profitability.

There are hundreds of businesses that offer dance competition experiences. You or I could start one at any moment, on any given day. They range from the rare nonprofits to the much more common for-profit sector.

Production values range from nonexistent to minimalist to over the top. In that regard, the industry is a lot like a theme park: you can find offerings ranging from backwoods, small competitions (like carnivals in parking lots) to mega-competitive events (like the largest, most successful theme parks).

Because clients are spending a lot of money for every type of event, they have a difficult time discerning the branding differentiation, and the mega-competitions maintain an upper hand on the market. Parents and students want the lighting rig, booming music, fog, and merchandise areas. Why? It affirms their investment in the value of the expense.

At a smaller event I attended, the judges sat in the balcony with their socked feet perched over the edge. The dance terminology on their critique sheets was handwritten and misspelled (plié was listed as pile), and to this day, I wonder if they watched any of our routines.

On another occasion, I volunteered as the committee chair for a nonprofit competition that uses entry fees to return to students in the form of scholarship dollars for continuing dance education. This mission is much more aligned to my values, and I was excited to join a team of educators in producing a simplified event. Parents were outraged at the minimalistic setup. Even with an explanation of the mission of the organization, they could not see past what they were used to expecting. Simply stated: scholarship and educational dollars were not as alluring as flashy setups with big names. The facade matters.

The big events are not utopic by any stretch of the imagination. At a mega-event that no longer exists, it was routine for the instructors to show up late with their sunglasses on, visibly exhausted from late nights of partying and seeming slightly annoyed by their responsibilities for the event. In my research, it seems this is still the case per an anonymous employee feedback listed in 2017 on Glassdoor under "Advice to Management" for Break the Floor Productions, the largest producer of competitive/convention events:

> "Your tours are geared for children and families, so having workers wanting to get blasted every tour stop and show up to work drunk, hungover, beyond late or worse, sends a terrible message."

The owner of Break the Floor responded in late 2019 with:

*"Thanks for your feedback. We have recently hired new management and are doing our best to improve some of the things you mentioned."*[3]

The behavior isn't frowned upon. It's ingrained in the culture. At Showstopper, teachers are handed cheap, branded bottles of wine in their welcome packets. Doesn't it seem odd (and somewhat inappropriate) for instructors and coaches to receive event-endorsed alcohol at a children's extracurricular event? Are coaches given pints of beer at the top of T-Ball games?

Adjudication systems are as individualized and varied as the owner(s) of the company. The "judges" are an extension of the company's culture and have their own set of rules, expectations, and guidelines. Feedback methods may include written score sheets and audio or video critiques and feedback, which often focus on technical, creative, performance, and choreographic components. Events have great judges, and events have terrible judges. One critique may only say "Good job," while other critiques delve into the mechanics of the movement. All are priced the same, and consistency doesn't exist.

The actual scoring metric for any given routine is a crap-shoot. It may be a forward-facing, 100-point scale where

---

3    "Break The Floor Productions Reviews," Glassdoor, accessed April 24, 2020, https://www.
     glassdoor.com/Reviews/Break-The-Floor-Productions-Reviews-E897101.htm.

a 10-point scale is the only part that's used. Routines are scored to the hundredth of the point.

In addition to the fees incurred by the client, there's also the merchandise section: T-shirts, hoodies, stuffed animals, program books, performance photography and videography, and more sparkly knickknacks and doodads than you can possibly imagine.

My experience within this roller coaster ride of an industry represents several perspectives: as a trophy-hungry child, as a dancer in the late '90s and early 2000s, as a teacher in the mid-late 2000s, as a studio owner between 2009 and 2015, and as a competitive judge between 2010 and 2015.

## AS A TROPHY-HUNGRY CHILD

Growing up, I wanted a trophy more than anything. I was an overachieving, straight-A student, but I craved a souvenir of accomplishment like all the other kids. If the kids on the softball team were getting a trophy, I wanted one, too.

My first test in the trophy-earning market was in the Fairest of the Fair Contest at the Greene County Fair in Greeneville, Tennessee. I had a gorgeous (or, maybe hideous?), frilly, perfectly '90s gown and the curliest bangs and permed hair imaginable. Prior to the pageant, we completed a "getting to know you" survey, which included a blank for the contestant's favorite food.

As the girls paraded, I could hear their favorite foods being announced in the small backstage hallway: pizza, mac and cheese, hamburgers. When I made my debut to the stage, I hit all the staging marks and cringed when I heard my favorite food read aloud: salmon patties.

Ugh! I still cringe about writing that as my answer. I didn't have a passion for salmon patties. They were what I had for dinner the day I completed the survey. So weird. So uncool. I did not take home a trophy or a tiara that day, but I learned my brain did not gravitate to the forward-facing, popular answers for "favorite food." It seemed superfluous. It was also an early lesson that I wasn't meant to play this kind of game.

I can still remember the second glorious day that bookended my short-lived pageant career. I entered the Pre-Teen Tennessee contest in Knoxville, Tennessee, and title holders wore the most beautiful sashes and tiaras. We dined on chocolate-pudding parfaits as we practiced proper etiquette. I dreamed of wearing a sash and a tiara but wasn't destined for either. Instead, I received the trophy for "highest score on the general knowledgeability test." Seriously?!

My short-lived pageant career that spanned my tenth year

of life ended. I tossed the "knowledge trophy" in the corner and carried on, understanding that these menial events were not going to define the outcome of my success.

At the time, I didn't understand how cool it is to be smart, how unimportant it is for the public to know your favorite food, and how little trophies matter in the scheme of things.

## AS A DANCER

As a dancer, I always found competitions to be fun experiences. I was never a soloist; it was always about the group camaraderie. I also wasn't the best technician. I had to work (really) hard to be a part of the group, and I took my hard work very seriously. I practiced at home, constantly created my own routines, and aimed to bring my best to the group effort.

I participated in a pre-social media world. My tenure as a competitive dancer featured honorable-mention ribbons and the occasional plaque of victory. A few times, I was cut out of sections of routines because I couldn't master the turn sequence. By cut out, I mean I ran off stage for the section and rejoined when the section ended. For all practical purposes, I was a "loser" at dance competitions.

So, what did I gain? The recognition never mattered to me; it was about travel, growth, and experiences. It was about the camaraderie and personal improvement. When my dance friends and I went on a two-week trip to Los Angeles, the group voted for me as the "Most Congenial." That handmade piece of construction paper meant more to me than any other dance competition adjudication I received. It was genuine and heartfelt. I feel like dance has given me a second family in several different iterations.

The entire participatory experience fueled my fire to hustle more and work harder. I adored my teachers and teammates and wanted to spend as much time with them as possible in adventurous and exciting new cities. I can tell you our routines, the people who were involved, the cities that we visited, the shows we performed, and the memories we made. Do you know what I can't remember? Our competition scores.

This was the purest perception of the industry I experienced, and I am grateful for this opportunity because I know that many of my students who once participated likely had some iteration of their own positive experience.

## AS A TEACHER

After high school, I had to figure out how I was going to keep dance in my life. I did not make the dance company at NC State and was not hired the first few times I applied to be a dance instructor. Hello, rejection!

When I was finally hired to teach, I was ready and determined to be the BEST dance teacher I could possibly be. To be a strong teacher, you must be a lifelong student. In and out of the classroom, I committed to learning as much as I possibly could about technique, style, history, and educational and behavioral classroom strategies. I wanted to know everything possible that would improve my success in this role.

As a teacher, I loved competitions because it was a medium to showcase my work. I was young with a hungry ego (late teens–early twenties) and was ready to get to business. I'd been choreographing in my bedroom for decades. I wanted to get a piece in front of some judges! As the wins rolled in, I found certain competitive recognitions validated my place in an industry that had initially rejected me.

Best choreography recognition?

Great!

I also loved the camaraderie. Traveling and enjoying meals with my colleagues was fun. The stakes were low—I could come in, get out, and have a great time. And I was good at it.

This was also when I first noticed the tension competitions could create—between students and between staff. People envied and craved success, even in its rawest, beginner form.

## AS A STUDIO OWNER

As a young and ambitious new studio owner, I was excited about the opportunity to build and create memorable, competitive experiences for my own tribe. I had waited for this moment my entire life!

When we had a competitive dance program, the sales points were:

- Opportunity to perform
- Experience of being a part of team
- Life-oriented skills (goal achievement)
- Confidence building through creativity

At some point in our path, these sales points were abandoned, and the focus became entangled in winning. Ultimately, it detracted from the success of my overall business and offered a valuable learning experience. It also reiterated the importance of maintaining corporate culture and brand consistency, even when there's pushback.

## AS A COMPETITIVE JUDGE

When I think back on my days of judging dance competitions, I easily spent months of my life watching routines. I watched studios all around the country pour their hearts on stage every weekend. I would judge for thirty-five to forty hours and fly back to my fifty to sixty-hour work week. Healthy work-life balance? Absolutely not.

I witnessed mega-studios entering hundreds of routines in a weekend. Being immersed as an outsider with no "skin in the game" gave me insight and wisdom I could not accrue in my other roles as a business owner, educator, and choreographer. I saw smaller schools trying to find validation on stage. I met amazing people who are so talented and passionate about this art. I stayed in nice hotels and horrible hotels and took flights at the most ungodly hours of the day.

I discovered the inside business of the competitive dance industry and watched as it impacted my studios. During this period, I kept thinking a change would happen, that someone would realize the opportunity to make it better. Instead, the machine keeps cranking, and the majority continue to participate.

These participatory roles, spanning three decades, provided unique perspectives on a variety of "rides" within the competitive dance industry. In my heart, I held the best memories. In my head, I could see the detriment it was starting to create for my studio...and it forced me to reflect on how all of this began.

When my studio started participating in the competitive industry, we started from the beginning. We did not inherit trained dancers, so we built from the ground up. If you've been there, you know it's not easy. It requires time, patience, and hard work.

In the early years, we would receive second place and be the only routine in the category (yes! that's a possibility). Emotions ranged from wanting to fist-pump in enthusiasm to wanting to crawl under the auditorium seats. We were raw and learning together. It was frustrating, but it was thrilling. The challenge seemed fun.

During this period of discovery, we recognized that our youngest dancers were our greatest opportunity since they were trained in-house and did not come with the baggage of "studio hoppers" (a family who travels from studio to studio in hopes of finding something that may or may not exist) or people looking for a "quick win" (a mentality that never interested me).

Once the younger students started receiving recognition, we gained more traction and interest in our competitive opportunities. Our four-year-olds were winning Highest Score of the Day! We had students winning "titles" (Mister and Junior Miss Star Glitz!), and people were delighted about our newfound competitive dance success. Heads turned toward us, and it infused an aura of excitement and intrigue.

There's a lot of baggage and expectation that comes with

being a "winner." People have a harder time understanding losses, and the focus on the win becomes all-consuming.

Over the years, I've considered why this attitude develops.

1. People are investing lots of time.
2. People are investing lots of money.
3. People expect a tangible, positive (winning) outcome for their investment.
4. People are placing an extreme valuation on the representation of the labels that are relatively meaningless within the construct of this environment.
5. Because of the investment, meaning is essential in justifying the participatory sacrifice.

At hypercompetitive dance studios, parents may spend upwards of $15,000 per semester or $25,000 per season on team-based training, choreography, costumes, travel, and entry fees. That's an extreme example, but it happens, and it happens more frequently than you might imagine. When I asked a friend from outside the industry what they'd expect for that amount, without hesitation, they said, "A win."

Parents take second mortgages on their homes to facilitate their child's winning dreams.

Emmy-winning choreographers are recruited to set dancers' multiple solos year after year.

Families are separated for extreme periods of time as they pursue their competitive dance conquests. School is placed on the back burner.

The addiction to winning is real, and once a family enters the cycle, there's reputability, stakes, and judgment on the line. They are attending these events with friends, neighbors, and their immediate community. Support can quickly shift to envy.

When this level of expectation is tied to the educational process of a developing child's extracurricular activity, it becomes toxic, damaging, and counterintuitive to what these activities should represent. Plus, the competitive dance scene is inconsistent and unpredictable. How do you justify or value a win versus a loss when a child is on an educational journey?

Humans want to win. It feels good and affirms their work and investment.

There's nothing wrong with a competitive desire to achieve excellence.

When pursuing victory, it is important to consider the stakes of the win:

- What does this win represent?

- What did this win cost?
- Is the win being sought for the right reasons?
- In a series of wins, how does the win differentiate?
- Is the win the only metric being used for personal progress?
- Are the wins meaningful to personal growth in one year, five years, or ten years?

If the product of the win is valued over the process of the journey, the desire to win is rooted in the wrong place. Experience is key for any craft and any level of accomplishment.

For example, if you book a Broadway show because of the expectation of winning a Tony Award, you are working for the win versus working for the vehicle of passion and purpose.

Tom Cruise has not won an Oscar. He's still making movies.

Numerous publishers rejected J. K. Rowling. Harry Potter is a household name.

Dan Marino never won a Superbowl. He's one of the greatest NFL Quarterbacks of all time.

Jennifer Hudson didn't win American Idol. She's one of the best voices to ever grace the show.

Notoriety is relative.

The meaning, passion, and purpose behind the process of the art is what should take priority.

Like roller coasters, the entertainment industry is full of hills and valleys. It is the highest of highs and the lowest of lows. Winning is never guaranteed (heck, in the professional world, working is not even guaranteed), so the love, discipline, and hustle must be instilled for the right reasons.

The peak of our success in the competitive dance industry marked the most miserable I'd ever felt. As we received a Champion of Champions Award in Orlando in Summer 2014, I looked at a girlfriend and asked if winning dance competitions would eventually feel better. Her response left me in chills: "Do you want me to tell you it will?"

With the hype and our reputation increasing, I threw myself into the work and hit pause on my emotions and personal feelings. I opened a second studio location and received a 40 Under 40 Recognition that enabled me to go to a three-day executive coaching retreat that proved to be painfully intense.

At the retreat, I was forced to pause.

During three days of meditation, digital deprivation, self-discovery, and conversation, I realized I had silenced my voice and neglected my own emotions and feelings for the sake of perceived societal expectations in my field (which mirrored the same imposter syndrome experience I had in college).

I was overwhelmed, slightly terrified, and marginally excited/empowered at the amount of work I needed to do—for myself and for the studio. At the heart of the conflict was the studios' participation in the competitive dance industry. I ugly-cried the entire way home because I wasn't sure where to start.

When I casually mentioned the idea of transitioning our program to noncompetitive to a valued client, their response was simple: "If you do that, we'll quit and find another studio."

This was going to be a tremendous, uphill battle.

At that moment, I knew client loyalty was no longer connected to the hours of training I was providing or the relationships I was building. Instead, it was aggressively earmarked to achieve coveted trophies and fleeting social media fame at any cost.

How often do we push our personal needs and feelings to the back burner because they're inconvenient or don't meet the expectations of someone else? Identifying the ins and outs of emotions is tough. You should pursue what feels right to you even if it contradicts the societal or industrial standard.

The journey I was about to begin was not going to be short or easy. It had to be an intentional phase of self-discovery. I knew we could merge passionate and purposeful artistic work that resulted in meaningful wins and recognitions as a collective team.

The "trophy" may come in the form of:

- Impact or influence
- Personal growth
- Transformation

The "trophy" should not come at the expense of:

- Relationships
- Emotional or physical well-being
- Basic ethical principles

This thought process requires consistency in intention and communication.

As a player in the children's extracurricular market, setting accurate guidelines and intentional expectations is key in framing the educational process and paving the baseline for our students' success.

As a business, our competitors are not other dance studios. Rather, we compete with literally anything else a child may choose to do instead of dance (soccer, voice, piano, gymnastics, staying at home and watching TV, playing with their friends). The value in the experience is paramount, and when the competitive piece was a part of our dance program, we were not reaching the overall value I envisioned.

I became disillusioned with the facade of the competitive dance industry as it was presented to the public. I felt as though I was looking behind the Wizard's curtain in *The Wizard of Oz*. While I tried to maintain enthusiasm about our experience-oriented participation, I couldn't help but acknowledge this gut feeling that something didn't feel right. The competitive dance industry roller coaster was slowly starting to feel like it was derailing, and I wanted off the ride.

I gave myself two (long) years to observe and affirm my feelings as well as reflect on our experiences. This was important because in the secular dance industry (nonconservatory and nonclassical), the competitive component is often tied to the perceived success of the organization, even if the competitive piece represents a minority percentage of the studio's overall population.

As expected, my feelings of discontent increased. It was hard to patiently and professionally navigate my feelings during this "holding period." Change is a process.

Change does not arrive wrapped in a box with a pretty bow. In a society that is centered around instant gratification, the expectation of fast, ceremonious, and hypersuccessful change is one of the greatest roadblocks we have in reaching our fullest potential and success as corporations and individuals. A story that's made for a movie typically does not happen overnight.

The counterargument insists it is easier to be complacent. Why change when what you are doing is working? Change is a risk. There are unknowns. It's a gamble. It is amazing how miserable people allow themselves to feel because of the fear of change. It can be personally and professionally paralyzing.

As I started warming up to the idea of radical change, I kept wondering, what would I do if the competitive industry imploded tomorrow?

If it did not exist, how would I create opportunities for my students?

I questioned why we allow a piece of our market to be hyperreliant on an industry that is out of our control. Were we puppets to their falsities? By endorsing this industry, was I creating a disservice for my clients?

The stakes were not low. I had two commercial leases in a

major metro area, a reputation in the industry, and a rapport with clients. Based on my initial survey, I knew we were poised to lose some key, highly connected, and highly valued stakeholders if we made the change.

That's scary stuff.

If you've ever felt one thousand and one questions running through your head, I can relate. At the crossroads of change, there's typically a motivator moment, a gentle nudge that leaves you feeling unsettled.

My motivator moment happened when competitions started giving "kindness" awards.

In revisiting this recognition, the "Competition Kindness" award is described as:

> "an initiative started to encourage dancers, studio owners, teachers, and parents to add value to the experience of all dancers while they train, perform and compete. The ability to be kind and supportive to someone who shares the same passion as you is something that helps us all grow and be better people, not only at competitions, but in life."[4]

On paper, this recognition does not sound terrible. It sounds

4    "Competition Kindness," StarQuest, accessed April 24, 2020, https://www.starquestdance.com/competition-kindness-2/.

very accurate and idealistic, like the outward-facing perception of dance competition participation. Yes! We should all be nice to each other.

I appreciate and applaud the recognition of a needed industry correction. Clearly, there was a tipping point that pushed the need for this level of dialogue. But does respect, kindness, and positive human interaction require a trophy? I always understood it as a basic human trait—an expectation instead of an award. This preserves authenticity and discourages disingenuous or contrived behavior.

Around the same time, on a late Sunday night in December, I received a seemingly kind resignation letter from one of my instructors:

> "I wanted to let you know that I will not be returning to Stage Door Dance in the spring.
>
> I truly apologize if this timing is inconvenient for you. I am very sad and I have enjoyed my time working with you and teaching the students. At this point in my life with my changes on the horizon, it is the right decision for me and for the studio.
>
> I sincerely appreciate how flexible you have been at accommodating my schedule over these past years. I cannot thank you enough for the opportunity to get to know you and teach for you."

I include the text of this note because, like the Competition Kindness Award, this did not sound terrible. Lives change, and people come and go. Initially, I did not assume this situation would be any different. Remember when I mentioned my naive optimism?

The kindness award was a response to backstage bullying and unfavorable behaviors on the part of students, teachers, and parents that infiltrated the competitive industry. While the behaviors were rampant, they were also impossible to wrangle and address. The positive reinforcement was intended to redirect the behaviors. However, respect should be a basic human right, not an awarded accomplishment. Little did I know the same behavior was happening in my backyard, too.

The instructor who resigned? She sent an entirely different, secret recruitment letter to the parents of selective students from my studio for her own competitive dance programming and personal gain. She had a major "in it to win it" attitude, and several of our intensely competitive families ruthlessly admired her drive. It didn't stop at recruiting students for her dance gain—she also invited six out of the twelve students on our Mini Competition Team to be flower girls in her wedding.

The kindness award juxtaposed with the resignation letter were the major motivators I needed to acknowledge change as a necessity. Both situations were facades to bigger problems that the competitive dance industry rampantly fuels, particularly regarding ethics. It was now immediately impacting the studios, and I missed when it felt like a happy place. Before it would get better, it would get much worse.

Late one Tuesday night, Jaimie, a former studio mom who also happens to be one of my best friends, rushed back into the studio and told me she felt something bad was happening. She was borderline panicked. I didn't buy into it and assured her everything was going to be okay. I believed what was in front of me, which was a terrible miscalculation.

A week or two later, the five- to seven-year-old students started telling our other instructors about their secret meetings and opportunities with the instructor who left our studio. Their parents instructed the students to keep the details "quiet," but children are honest and transparent.

When attempting to openly and honestly address the topic with my clients, they brazenly said, "They had a right to shop at Walmart or Target" and would approach their dance education in the same way. The shockwaves that rippled through our business were intense and daunting.

In the years since this transpired, I've been told there were meetings at hotels, at houses, and in client-owned businesses. They were competing new, secretly choreographed solos and forgetting the choreography they were learning as a part of their team. The toxicity was rampant, and nobody involved was immune to the impact.

As I tried to keep the businesses as consistent and steady as possible, the group that aligned with the former instructor quickly villainized me. At the same time, I had to address the feelings of anger, sadness, and discontent from the families who were ostracized from this special group.

When you have two parties so equivocally divided, how do you find a middle ground?

This is the question we frequently ask in large-scale political or religious arenas.

Now, we were asking the same question for a divisiveness felt within a dance studio.

I knew the solution was on the outside of everything I had known. I had to respond versus react. This would prove to be the greatest test in leadership I have experienced. It was time to prepare for the transition as well as creatively implement and activate an exciting alternative option that would either make or break my business.

At North Carolina State University, we are taught to "think and do the extraordinary."

This was my chance.

The roller coaster of a ride with dance competitions wasn't fun anymore. In fact, it was sickening, and I was ready to be done. It was flying off the tracks, and I was not okay with it.

We often stay involved with situations, people, and things for way too long because we are fearful of the unknown and because questioning the norm is exhausting. What if we consciously diverted our instincts to be excited about the opportunity for creating something new? Check in with your emotions; ask yourself the tough questions about why people linger in discomfort. The people and things that matter will still be with you—even after you choose to stop riding roller coasters, literally and metaphorically.

*Chapter 3*

# STAY ALERT

Going with the flow is easy. It requires way less work and thought. Yet, consider everything society wouldn't have if everyone decided to go with the flow. Particularly, think about what would happen if people decided to go with the flow when it is counterintuitive to their purpose and passion. Innovation and change may not impact everyone, but if we are all working toward improving our ecosystems in the best ways we can, impact will universally expand.

Growing up, every time a big change or opportunity was in front of me, I created a list of "pros" and "cons." It's elementary in concept, but I still do this and encourage my dancers to do the same when they are weighing options and decisions. Because I care so much about the performing arts and its lasting integrity, specifically its capabilities for empowering and inspiring children, it was exceptionally important to approach the impending change in our business with as much thoughtful information as possible.

Radical change is not the time to be flippant. The decision had to be considered from every angle to make sure I wasn't overly wrapped up in personal feelings, bias, and emotion. I needed to identify any "blind spots," so I started by creating a list of questionable perceptions/actualities of the competitive dance experience that were outside of the stress and conflict I was immediately feeling and directly experiencing. When I revisited this document for the book, I was shocked to see that there were nearly twenty major negative hindrances influencing my decision. That's a lot!

Some topics are surface-level observations, and some are much deeper. The feedback is a combination of external observation, client and staff feedback, and general industry conversation. Because there's minimal research or documentation on any of these topics, the ramifications and lasting impacts are still unknown.

## COMPETITIVE VERSUS RECREATIONAL

Growing up, I never noticed inclusivity versus exclusivity at dance, but when I started teaching in a more metropolitan area, I noticed a clear divide in the way students were labeled and treated as either recreational or competitive students. The differentiation in labeling clearly happened as the competitive component became a larger piece of dance studio operations.

This distinction feels unsettling because it projects a sense of importance upon the competitive students, while the recreational students are deemed as "lesser than." As educators, we have a calling to pour our full investment into all of our students in hopes that the skills and learning process will better the students' human condition.

When children study an extracurricular, their training should be high quality, regardless of whether a student opts to participate at a higher level. For example, if a child goes to swim lessons, the child should have proficiency and confidence in the water. If a child takes a dance class, there should be proficiency and confidence in skill, creativity, and confidence in presentation/performance.

Within the dance studio environment, there must be caution on how we label, treat, and perceive our students. Let's use our language to cultivate an environment of proficiency and inclusivity while recognizing that students will progress at different rates and may choose to train at different levels.

## DANCE MOMS

When *So You Think You Can Dance?* launched in 2005, it

brought a healthy competitive spirit for adult dancers that showcased a variety of styles and creative, themed choreography. It was great exposure for the industry and reinvigorated the public interest in the art of dance. Younger dancers eagerly watched and were excited for their opportunity to one day audition for the show. The show's producer, Nigel Lythgoe, created the Dizzy Feet Foundation in 2009 and National Dance Day in 2010. This was all super productive and gained an incredible amount of positive media attention for dance!

Then, in 2011, all those positive, public-facing strides came to a screeching halt when the reality show *Dance Moms* emerged. One of my girlfriends was vetted for this show, and she knew from the outset it was going to be too controversial to touch. In its first two seasons, the show reached 200 million viewers,[5] bringing unprecedented mass attention to dance competitions for all the wrong reasons.

The competitive dance industry undoubtedly preyed upon this exposure.

Gary Pate of Starpower openly stated their registration numbers increased with studios intent upon beating the Abby Lee Dance Company. He also recognized, "People

---

5    Rachel Zar, "Sorting the Reality from the Reality TV with Abby Lee Miller," *Dance Teacher Magazine*, October 2012.

don't want to watch a goody-two-shoes dance teacher. They want to see dysfunction."[6]

Dysfunction is what they received: on screen and in real life.

As the show continued season after season, the following normalizations occurred:

- The acceptability of inappropriate routines, costumes, and behavior
- The exploitation of children for the sake of entertainment
- The "get it at any expense" trick-oriented mentality of choreography
- The extremely intense must-win attitude

Over the years, competitions have tiptoed away from affiliating their brand with *Dance Moms*. Dance Masters of America and StarQuest were two of the first to speak out against the show and its ethical dilemmas. If you dig a little deeper, there are countless articles about the misrepresentation of scoring and the staged "reality" components, as well as about more serious topics such as assault, tax evasion, and the detrimental impact and influence the show had on the competitive dance market.

---

6    Rachel Zar, "Sorting the Reality from the Reality TV with Abby Lee Miller," *Dance Teacher Magazine*, October 2012.

Abby Lee Miller trained some brilliantly successful performers and entertainers. If you combine her produced television persona in a hypercompetitive atmosphere with caricatures of stage moms, it creates a recipe for disaster. People see the environment and success as an aspiration. It becomes a requirement for success versus sheer entertainment.

In the show's early days, I was one of the 200 million viewers. It seemed so absurd and extreme to see this perception of my industry on television that it was nearly laughable. Then, it started feeling like my life was becoming this world. People would enter our studio asking for a "Dance Moms" experience.

The media and hype surrounding this show was intense, and the competitive spirit it fostered was counterproductive to the healthy development of a child as well as the overall environment of the competitive dance industry.

## THE HYPERSEXUALIZATION OF CHILDREN

The costumes. The music. The material and themes. Some of the moves. There is so much hypersexualization of female children in the competitive dance industry.

In a world of heightened sensitivity, I am astonished this topic has never gained traction in the mainstream media.

In 2010, there was a short burst of media frenzy surrounding a dance performed by young dancers to Beyonce's "Single Ladies." I revisited the video, which now has millions of views on YouTube. The comments are turned off, but the video snippet I referenced has 35,000 "thumbs up" and 9,600 "thumbs down," proving the divisiveness of the conversation.[7]

The dancers have strong technique and exceptional energy and commitment to their performance. However, the costumes and suggestive styling of some of the moves are grossly inappropriate for seven-year-old dancers. The parents defended the choice as completely appropriate.

An ABC News article featured perspectives from both sides:[8]

- One father argued that the routine was not intended for the masses and had been taken completely out of context. He felt it was a completely normal routine for children to perform.
- As a collective, the parents of the performers claimed they did this in the best interest of their children.

7   "Single Ladies Dance (7 years old-Original)," YouTube, May 15, 2010, https://www.youtube.com/
    watch?v=ir8BO4-7DkM.

8   John Berman, Sarah Netter, "Young Girls' 'Single Ladies' Dance Sparks Controversy
    on Internet," ABC News, May 14, 2010, https://abcnews.go.com/GMA/Parenting/
    girl-single-ladies-dance-sparks-controversy-internet/story?id=10644648.

- One viewer questioned the legality of showing children performing such suggestive moves.
- Another viewer argues that if (a viewer) feels the performers are doing anything wrong, they are imposing their own perverted views on the situation.

In modern society, it's sociologically fascinating how immediate infuriation gains traction. Equally fascinating is how quick we are to abandon an issue, moving on to the next outrage without any actual action addressing the situation. How do we keep turning our heads and allowing this level of thematic material to infiltrate performance space that features minor participants?

In 2013, I was asked to do a phone interview with a student completing a grad school project about the competitive dance circuit. Ironically, I took the interview while attending a national convention and competition in New Orleans. Assuming the article was for school research, I willingly offered a lot of candid insight. In November 2014, the content of the interview was shockingly published in *Bitch* magazine in an article entitled "Babes in Danceland: When Did Competitive Dance Get So Sexy?"[9]

Yikes.

---

9  "Babes in Danceland: When did competitive dance get so sexy?" *Bitchmedia*, November 21, 2014, https://www.bitchmedia.org/article/babes-in-danceland-competitive-dance-too-sexy.

I was mortified because this felt misaligned from my brand. I was still competing, and the article was showing up on page three when you Googled my name. The quotes and the general tone of the article were counterintuitive to everything I represented. I emailed, begging them to remove it. They refused, and I continued to freak out.

In retrospect, the interview captured some of my unsettled thoughts and observations that were weighing heavily on my mind. My reaction to the magazine was knee-jerk, a nervous response to the premature distribution of this type of information with my name attached.

My quotes included the following:

"The punishment for inappropriateness happens extremely infrequently on the competition circuit because each judge must agree..."

"In an artistic world, interpretation can certainly vary. Something I may find inappropriate, another judge might be perfectly fine with..."

"I am seeing a rise in 7- to 10-year-olds wearing revealing costumes like skimpy 'Band-Aid' tops and booty shorts. Although the onus may be partially on costuming companies, it is ultimately the teachers' responsibility to match the costume to both the concept of the dance and the age of the dancer."

*Bitch* magazine likely does not have a huge readership circulation, and nobody ever brought the article to my attention. In the moment, it worried me because I did not have a clearly defined alternative position. What would my peers think? I tend to shy away from extremist positions, and this felt so extreme. At that moment, I felt sick with discomfort.

Clearly, the discomfort laid in my words mismatching my actions.

I was a hypocrite.

I wish this conversation had developed a little more at the time, and I wish I had not felt so initially shy or uncomfortable about my position. I also wish I had not used the words *"Band-Aid" tops* or the word *onus*; both of those bother me to this day.

Side note: I now confirm all interview content and usage before providing it.

## "PENIS POINTS"

This terrible phrase is an incredibly crass assumption and label given to male dancers who quickly gain success in the competitive dance industry.

"Oh, he only won because of penis points."

"Their dance outplaced our dance because the judge gave them penis points."

It is reverse gender inequality. As a Southerner, I am particularly familiar and sensitive to common, albeit inaccurate, positioning that boys shouldn't dance. I have a major problem with anyone dissuading male participation or accomplishment in the field of dance.

Negativity should not be tied to gender-based participation. I saw it happen in the competitive dance space, and years later, I heard the dissuasion again when Lara Spencer challenged Prince George's participation in ballet on *Good Morning America*. I felt compelled to post the following on my social media on August 23, 2019.

"Hey Lara Spencer & Good Morning America:

Let's take a minute to discuss boys in ballet/dance from the educational perspective I've had after 11 years serving as the Owner/Artistic Director of Stage Door Dance Productions in Raleigh, North Carolina.

The boys I've collectively taught have two Tony awards, three Broadway shows, one national tour, a UNCSA high school education, a USC Glorya Kaufman School of Dance education, film and tv credits, and countless other accolades.

Let's also talk about the REAL impact of boys in dance:

I have a boy signing up to start class because his physical therapist believes it will help with his mild cerebral palsy.

I have a boy who was born with clubfoot that had to fight to learn how to walk and now he expresses himself with movement and ballet.

I've taught the boys at the Governor Morehead School for the Blind. One of those boys went on to UNC-Charlotte and is majoring in Dance. He is the first UNC-C dance student with a visual impairment and the university has worked with him to develop a "movement mentor" program.

I've witnessed the joy that dance brings to the boys at the Frankie Lemmon School and Development Center.

I've had the honor of teaching a young boy who lost his life way too soon from cancer and had the incredible privilege of working with him and his mom on a very special routine.

In the last 6 years, I've directed and/or choreographed 35 theatre productions in our area. I've watched teen to adult males give their all to learn choreography, including ballet, to create exceptional performances that make Raleigh an artistically rich area to live.

Let's take a moment and focus on how we can lift others up instead of tearing people down. I believe that dance is for all ages, all genders, and all levels of ability. We need to strip away this stigma and bullying that surrounds boys and dance, and instead, celebrate the many ways it can positively impact our students and our society!"

In a world that is constantly discussing equality, I am amazed and horrified at the preexisting gender disparities in the field of dance.

Donald O'Connor.

Gene Kelly.

Jerome Robbins.

Alvin Ailey.

Bob Fosse.

Patrick Swayze.

This is a small sampling of the male entertainers who inspired and delighted my love for the performing arts. Their talent is exceptional and their legacy is unparalleled. We need to make sure we are promoting dance in a way that encourages inclusion of any gender identity, so we do not isolate or ostracize a future great from participating in this art.

## LACK OF ORIGINAL MATERIAL

Originality in art is a philosophical issue. It's a deeper topic that requires lengthy conversation. Stealing choreography and repurposing it for the sake of winning dance competitions does not require conversation because it is blatantly wrong. I am shocked it even happens.

I encountered this firsthand when I discovered that a former instructor was finding all of her "inspiration" for choreography from a saved YouTube playlist on her personal account. When I pulled up the playlist, nearly every routine my students had performed was featured, only years earlier. Ethically, this felt incredibly wrong.

Why in the world would an artist sacrifice their ability to create for a chance to win? It is a misrepresentation of the art as well as a worrisome lesson to our students. Do we want them thinking that cheating or borrowing another's source material is the quick way to gain notoriety and achievement?

Do we discard our ability to grow as choreographers and artists because it is easier to win than it is to challenge our own creative intelligence? Is pressure from clients a driving force behind the fear of innovation and creativity within this medium?

## SKEWED ADJUDICATION

In the competitive dance industry, there's no regulation in scoring. People like the tangible results that can be found in basketball, gymnastics, or ice skating. How do you explain scoring when there is no standardized rubric or metric, and every event offers its own unique "pay to play" system?

Performing arts are interpretive to the eyes of the person experiencing the art, which encompasses the individual's values, experiences, education, beliefs, and preferences. Even when there are scoring recommendations presented to the judges within each competition, there's no way to guarantee consistency or even justification.

The industry used to score routines based on gold, silver, and bronze, a familiar system, like the Olympics. It was simple and straightforward; a few people labeled as winners, and everyone else went home and continued to work. As we evolved into a society of "everybody wins" and deserves a participation trophy, the scale shifted to ridiculously titled adjudications including titanium, platinum, crystal, and diamond as forced labels of top recognitions.

Adjudications now linger at the higher end of the scale,

and placement is coveted over the ranking. For example, if there are 140 Senior Division Solos in all different styles, the rankings may fall as follows: 15 Diamond Adjudications (the exceptional routines that will rank in the "Top 10"), 120 Platinum Adjudications (the average to above-average routines), and 5 High Gold Adjudications (the below-average routines). Notice: the below-average routines are deemed "High Gold"—the perfect representation of the skewed nature of the scale.

Every routine receives some type of insignia for their adjudication, and all performers are required to sit on stage together for each awards ceremony. Depending on the bell curve of the adjudications, you may know if you won a top position or if you fell into the very bottom of the rankings. Most of the performers fall somewhere in the middle, making the adjudications completely pointless and another superfluous reason to create unnecessary upset while wasting a significant amount of time.

Before moving into overall rankings, there may also be rankings by style (jazz, contemporary, tap, open, song and dance, etc.) and/or age (at some events, age may be broken down within a year of life [7-7.49 years old and 7.5-7.99 years old] to further spread the wealth).

Then, there's the divisional rankings, which is the moment most anticipate. Divisional rankings are where the "Top

However Many" are announced within the division. The number of rankings is determined based on the number of entries in the category. For example, Top 5 Mini Small Groups, Top 25 Senior Solos, Top 3 Teen Line, etc. Rankings may tie (yes, there can be three- and four-way ties for first place), which can create even further challenges and explanations for the scoring process. If you're the only routine in the category, you (most likely) win first place!

One or two times per event they will recognize the "best of" series (highest score of the day, best choreography, most creative, etc.). These are the most coveted awards, and they are typically recognized within two primary age breakdowns: 12 and Under and 13 and Over.

Side note: Beyond awards for dance, many competitions have a (paid) photogenic category, which feels so regressive for modern society. How do children feel receiving criticism about their outward appearance? While the photographic feedback is usually intended for the photographer, it directly impacts the participating child. It also has nothing to do with dance.

If you are confused about the insane number of awards, welcome to the club.

The awards distribution process is designed to be confusing, fast, and abundant.

In addition to adjudications and placements, there are also special awards. Special awards are generally given to the exceptional or nonexceptional routines. They may be for on-stage projection of personality, costuming, or truly exceptional technique. If you closely watch an awards ceremony, you can always tell if the recognition is going to an exceptional or nonexceptional routine. We once won a special award for music editing for using the song "Like It's Quidditch" (a Harry Potter-themed parody of "Like a G6"). That's an example of a nonexceptional special award.

At the end of an awards ceremony, a dancer can walk away with multiple pins, ribbons, dog tags, license plates, banners, trophies, or other forms of insignia to capture their weekend wins. Their arms are overflowing with collateral, and trophies are sometimes taller than the dancers themselves. Because the awards system is watered down, it can be hard to navigate who won what or why. There's no logic behind it. The modus operandi of the competition: keep the participants happy so they'll continue coming back for more.

## WHO GETS THE GLORY?

In the awards ceremony, our studio always assigned rotational spokespeople for different routines so everyone could practice their public-speaking skills. The students had a script and were instructed to credit "the staff at Stage Door

Dance" if they were asked about their teachers or choreographers. This answer was designed to enhance the feeling of community and collaboration instead of divisiveness.

With the plethora of insignia, there's usually one piece of hardware that's the center point of group routines. For example, if a small group has six participants, they'll receive a trophy for the group (intended for the studio) and six ribbons for each individual student. We always experienced arguments regarding who was going to retrieve the trophy, hold the trophy, ride in the car with trophy, etc. The conflict was not isolated to our dancers; it involved some of the parents, too.

The value that was placed on the trophy was mind-blowing. Instead of cherishing the memory, the opportunity, the experience, or the feedback, it was all about the item that marked the win.

I never wanted a studio covered in trophies because I feel that falsely represents the educational presence of a training facility. What did the "glory" even represent?

## LEVELS

Many of the competitions have levels, which are intended to separate competitors based on their experience and ability. In theory, the concept enables a gateway to the experience for new participants. Since the levels are not enforced at events, many studios use them to spread out their dancers so they aren't competing directly against each other (if they can help it). This way, they "win" more. Why does this happen? It keeps the parents happy!

During our competitive tenure, we almost always competed at the highest level. My opinion was, why pay to play unless you are pushing yourself to the top? When other studios were taking advantage of entering their routines in multiple levels (more trophies! more overalls!), it made it hard to explain our method to the parents of our competitive dancers.

In modern parenting culture, it seems much easier for a parent to walk out the door with a happy child, trophy in hand. Otherwise, there are negative emotions to address and deeper conversations to have. As a part of the cycle, when negative emotions arise and the child is displeased or unhappy, it becomes the studio's fault versus an opportunity for collaborative conversation and improvement between the parent, dancer, and studio. Parents prefer their child winning an overall trophy in a novice category (even if they aren't a novice) versus competing at the highest level.

This pattern expands beyond the dance industry. We are seeing it in education and extracurriculars, and the concern lies in the students' ability to prioritize experiences in a way that fosters adaptability and resilience. Manipulating the system may be a short-term victory, but it robs the student of necessary skills and experiences for long-term success.

## CONFLICTS OF INTEREST

Several competitions/conventions allow their faculty to choreograph for students who compete in their events. The larger studios that pay the most typically benefit from these relationships because the guest artist fees are significant.

The conversation of bias or conflict of interest has never been straightforwardly mentioned, but it undoubtedly exists. How can you refrain from advocating for something in which you have direct, immediate involvement and a vested interest? If you've produced quality work and you see it on stage, you should want it to win. Yet, you're also working for a conglomerate where you are supposed to be judging everything fairly, on an even plane. It's tough, and there's no way it can be fair.

Beyond judging one's own choreography, we have attended events with former employees on the judging panel. This is incredibly uncomfortable for all parties. It also indicates the competition's lack of vetting and client knowledge.

Nepotism is rampant in the competitive dance scene, which adds another complicated layer to the perception of participation. Parents often do not realize how interconnected relationships can be. Sometimes, when they realize the opportunity for interconnectivity, they seek ways to take advantage of it. This may include circumventing professional courtesy in communication, "trash talking" to affiliates from other studios, and directly questioning judges about their decisions.

All are unnecessary roadblocks to a successful and fair experience.

## THE RISE OF SOCIAL MEDIA
### ACCESSIBILITY TO INFORMATION

Social media creates unprecedented accessibility to dance videos. Routines and skills are available at your fingertips. "Tricks" are often featured; the amount of time/training it took to achieve the "trick" is not. This culture shift promotes product over process.

When the competitive dance industry is interjected into this equation, it means that clients can demand that a turn series, acrobatic skill, or progressive sequence be taught or mastered in an unrealistic and potentially unsafe amount of time. The educational journey and process is not honored; instead, it is stifled for the prospect of recognition.

One time, I had a few parents from a couple of hours away

reach out. They were from a smaller, rural studio, and the owner recommended supplemental training for the dancers to achieve their competitive goals. They heard I was a reputable technician and wanted their dancers to learn a complicated turn series to infuse into their competitive routines.

Could I teach it to them? Yes. But they were not ready to learn it. Instead, we had to focus on strengthening, ballet foundations, body alignment, and basic anatomical awareness before they were ready to begin working on their turn execution.

This was the beginning of a seven-year relationship with the families because the parents understood the educational process and wanted it for their children. That's a rarity. Their complete understanding, value, and trust in the process versus the product was refreshing. The one dancer who stayed with me the entire time is continuing her performance success in college.

When we educate and establish mutual partnerships, we thrive. Hard work pays off—there's no substitute for it.

Social media does not educate; it flaunts. Often, parents and dancers become so tied to a quick win, they lose sight of the power of the process. The process builds tenacity, discipline, work ethic, adaptability, and resilience. Digital accessibility has the potential to undermine the power of these character attributes.

## EXPLOITATION OF PRETEEN BRAND AMBASSADORS

Preteen and teen competitive dancers are used on social media to sell products. These dancers amass a significant following and have professional photo shoots featuring clothing and products that other dancers may want to wear.

The poses are often sultry. The clothing is typically minimal. Bra tops and brief or booty shorts are the norm. In order to promote brands, the account must stay public, inviting commentary and inappropriate remarks from the general public. In the profile bio, it will usually say "Mom Monitored," but does "Mom Monitored" limit the potentially negative impact of suggestive photos and/or the gross or inappropriate comments?

A typical post or report will direct readers to "follow" a certain site for access to promotions, deals, and secret sales. When you go to the main feed, you see tons of children in posed photos for their product. Has social media made us so desensitized to this trend that we are no longer looking out for the well-being of children?

Corporate accountability needs to be addressed. Would this form of advertising be permissible on a billboard in

Times Square? Absolutely not. We need to stop permitting the manipulation of children and their access to social media platforms for inappropriate corporate gain.

Outside of corporate accountability, what are the larger implications of suggestive preteen photography as it relates to body confidence, self-image, and personal identity as the children continue to navigate adolescence? Lindsey Giller, a clinical psychologist specializing in youth and young adults with mood disorders at the Child Mind Institute, notes, "Through likes and follows, teens are getting actual data on how much people like them and their appearance." Constant social media use can lead to anxiety, poor self-esteem, insecurity, and sadness in teens.[10]

Is this extension of the competitive dance industry confusing commercial exploitation as an appearance-based "win"?

## CYBERBULLYING AND PASSIVE EXCLUSION

With social media, teens can engage in cyberbullying and passive exclusion. This can happen without competitive stakes, so when the competitive piece is added, it undoubtedly intensifies.

---

10  Leah Shafer, "Social Media and Teen Anxiety," Usable Knowledge: Relevant Research for Today's Educators from Harvard Graduate School of Education, December 2017. https://www.gse.harvard.edu/news/uk/17/12/social-media-and-teen-anxiety

Cyberbullying actions may range from saying inappropriate things that would never be spoken in a person-to-person interaction to editing a person out of a photo or video. The hurt is real, and the understanding of the digital reality versus the actual reality is very blurred and misunderstood.

Whether the action is a snarky comment on a missed/imperfect move, poor song choice, routine placement, costume design, a ranking, or a misinterpreted situation, the falsely guarded, privatized world of Snapchats, chat boards, and other forms of passive media can be alarming.

Bullying is more prevalent than any of us would like to acknowledge. It happened to my students one spring at a major competition and convention in Greenville, North Carolina. We had a small group who performed a routine to "God Help the Outcasts" from *The Hunchback of Notre Dame.* It was a younger group, newer in their competitive experience. Because of the competition's scheduling, the dancers didn't have time to remove some of their eye makeup from a previously performed musical theatre routine. I like for things to run on schedule, so instead of holding up the competition with an extended makeup/costume change, we decided to leave it on for the performance.

One of the competition's "Outstanding Dancers" (a top honor) took to Twitter to share how laughable the group looked dancing to a sad, expressive song with theatrical makeup. Not only was this person making comments about our students and our studio; he was making equally disturbing, negative comments about other studios and students attending this event in real time through Twitter.

The saddest part? Bullying is not isolated to students. I've seen participating instructors, parents, and even adjudicators make ridiculously snide and passive remarks online.

## DISCOVERY

Social media as a platform for discovery is almost always hurtful.

I discovered a student had replaced their solo featuring my choreography with choreography from instructors at a different studio in a different state. The student was tagged as a featured student at the new studio. Screenshot after screenshot flooded my phone.

More surprising? The owners of the new studio actively recruited this student to train with them after observing successful performances at dance competitions. When I started exploring the situation, my student was not the first recruit training with them. This pattern of recruitment was habitual.

In other sports, at all levels, there are tampering rules. In the competitive dance industry, that doesn't exist. Even the rules that are published are not enforced.

That same season, I discovered a different student was secretly performing a new solo at competitions under a different studio name. The student was forgetting her set solo, which seemed unusual for this child. I started looking around and found the new solo on the results page of a competition. When I approached the parents with this information, they refused to have a conversation about their actions and left.

Both students have now trained with a myriad of dance studios and instructors. While I've lost touch with both, the way the scenarios were handled is what is most hurtful. Transparency and communication are key, and when deceit happens online, it destroys professional relationships and mangles trust.

Does the burden of responsibility fall on the dance teachers, the parents of dancers, or the competitive dance industry, which serves as a catalyst for this type of rogue, Wild West behavior?

## THERE IS NO "I" IN TEAM

While the team mentality is what the competitive community should breed, it doesn't. Instead, the "winning" individuals tend to become so self-focused that it breaks down the general construct of the group and the culture of the studio.

The "winning individuals" want to focus on solos and hand-selecting their dance partners. I've had parents blatantly tell me that group routines are a nuisance and a waste of time. Because the dance studio industry is also a business and not an Olympic training program, if you do not cater to the needs of the client, they leave.

I want to pause for a second because the ability to work collaboratively, in a team environment, is what pushes society forward. I would not be successful if I didn't have an amazing team standing behind me, and it worries me that the value of the group can be conveniently discarded for personal gain in this educational, extracurricular construct.

The leaving is easy when there are studios eager to recruit winning individuals. Like the winning individuals, there are studios that are equally enthusiastic about winning no matter the price—ethically or literally. Don't want to dance with your groups? Come to us. Only want to focus on your solo? Come to us. Want to perform at any and every event imaginable with minimal instructor guidance? Come to us.

There are supposedly rules to alleviate the epidemic of

studio-hopping, but like many of the other rules, they aren't enforced, and they can be easily circumnavigated. The truly sad part of this behavior is that the "winning individuals" are often seen as the leaders of the group and occasionally even as the leader within their aged cohort of the entire competitive dance industry.

In the extracurricular market, it is essential that we work together as parents, educators, and students to offer an ethical and productive training experience, especially when it involves cross-training and teams of educators. There's a right way and a wrong way to approach it, and unfortunately, the current trends affiliated with the competitive dance industry are predominantly aligned with the wrong approach.

## TOPICAL ROUTINES

The darkness of routines at dance competitions can be intense. It is hard to decipher if the material is coming from a place of education/storytelling or an emotionally manipulative strategy designed for winning.

Regardless, in an environment designed for children, it can be incredibly unsettling for audience members to watch routines about shootings, abuse, depression, and suicide. Is art designed to prompt conversation? Of course! However, there's an appropriate medium for it,

Parents should not feel uncomfortable watching routines with their children at dance competitions. I remember a parent from our studio covering the eyes of her six-year-old at a dance competition because the routine on stage was so dark and sexually suggestive.

Similarly, minors should not be expected to perform routines that are topically intense. Hard topics require tough conversations, which require careful, developmentally appropriate navigation and parental involvement.

Let's nurture and cultivate the creativity of our dancers in a positive, uplifting way. There's enough heaviness in life without it existing in this space, too.

## FORMULAIC PAY TO PLAY

In watching categories at dance competitions, you'll see there's a lot of dances that are similarly styled. Beyond blatantly stealing choreography, this happens because one dancer or style will consistently win, and then the other dancers begin imitating the choreography or using a popular song that's desperately begging for reprieve.

Consider the following scenarios:

- If ten senior contemporary solos are performed to "Can't Help Falling in Love" by Haley Reinhart (because dance competitions love an acoustic cover) in one weekend, how can a judge score solo number eight with the same freshness and clarity as solo number one?

· If there are four regional competitions in a season and there are two or three productions to "A Little Party Never Killed Nobody" by Fergie at each event, your studio clients may question your creative ability because everyone else is performing the same thing as your studio. If you don't win first place and the big kahuna of the weekend award, they'll question if your production might have scored better if a different song/theme/costume/choreography was chosen.

When choreography and performance become win-driven versus performance-driven, we lack innovation, emotion, and storytelling in the art. We create routine fatigue. Routine fatigue emerges as a by-product of duplication versus creation. Creating is a risk. There's no guarantee or likelihood a new, innovative style will receive strong accolades; yet, creativity is a necessity in advancing the art and advancing the industry.

If you look at musical theatre choreography, the advancement of styles from Jerome Robbins (*West Side Story)* to Bob Fosse *(Cabaret)* to Michael Bennett *(A Chorus Line)* to Andy Blankenbuehler *(Hamilton)* are unique, diverse, and exciting. This is a very limited scope and comparison, but the uniqueness is there. When watching their styles, you're captivated, engrossed, and excited at the movement combined with their storytelling capabilities.

Are the structure and expectations of the competitive dance industry limiting our creative freedoms and stifling our art? If you take the construct of the competitive environment away and perform for the sake and power of performing, there's freedom in choice, in growth, and in technical development as artists for the right reasons.

## THE DEVALUATION OF ACADEMICS

Our studio culture has always valued academics. I received the Park Scholarship at North Carolina State University, a full, merit-based academic scholarship for my undergraduate degree. I would not have achieved this without valuing academics in my educational journey.

My staff are also very accomplished in their undergraduate and graduate work, and our alumni are doing very smart, accomplished things in a variety of fields. Clients appreciate this component of our culture—we love and encourage smart dancers!

Toward the end of our competitive tenure, dance competitions started scheduling events and routines during the day on Friday, or sometimes beginning as early as Thursday evening. I would feel so stressed receiving this information because it placed an immense strain on our studio families. I knew they were going to be really upset and inconvenienced. We would receive the final schedule one or two weeks in advance, which didn't leave a lot of time for planning. Children were missing school, parents were missing work, dance instructors were missing their classes. Our ecosystem was off-balance and annoyed.

In January 2015, we attended an event in Richmond, Virginia. The schedule was released a week in advance, and parents were irate (at me) for the early morning start time.

Some emails I received:

> "I think it is absolutely ridiculous that these organizations can't have a better idea of start time until one week prior to the event..."

> "I tried getting a hotel room, but the rate is $279 for Thursday. The overflow hotel is sold out. If I knew we had that early of a call time, I would have booked accordingly, not to mention my daughter has a half-day field trip on Friday..."

> "What is a placement adjudication? Hope that means she can dance later as missing college classes is really not a great option!"

On one occasion, a student had a required test on Friday.

She could not make her solo routine that was scheduled on Friday, during the day. The competition would not move her time or offer a refund. I personally gave the family a refund (at a loss to the business), but the mother's upset feelings were not directed toward the competition; they were directed toward me.

Who can blame them? It genuinely seems ridiculous to expect families to abandon their commitments and routine at the last minute for the sake of a dance competition for which they are paying exorbitant prices to participate.

## EVENT DECORUM

If teaching, practicing, and encouraging theatre etiquette is a goal of a performance-based arts education, the competitive dance environment does not provide an appropriate setting.

People are constantly in and out of the performance area. Multiple times, events stop to request the audience to be quiet and respect the performers. One time, I was judging, and the noise immediately behind me was so loud and distracting that I could hardly focus on the routine on stage. Bottom line: if the routine isn't applicable to them, audience members don't care.

For routines that matter to audience members, it is not

unusual to see cowbells, boisterous yelling, and studio chants. The larger studios show up. Everyone knows who they are. A small routine from a studio with a small competitive team may hardly receive any applause, whereas a small routine from a studio with a large competitive team will receive gladiator-level applause. You can tell a student all day that the amount of applause they receive does not matter. But how do you think they feel when they hear the gladiator-level applause and it doesn't happen for them?

The awards ceremony is equally eye-opening. Students wander on the stage in their pajamas, most of them on their phones and not really paying attention. Invested audience members loudly shush those around them so they can anticipate their child's chance at victory.

As awards are read, parents will often shout:

"That's not right!"

"We can't hear you!"

"That's surprising!"

"What was that special award again?"

The backstage area is similarly chaotic. After rolling in custom, blinged-out Dream Duffels—pricey $300+ luggage designed especially for the competition—dancers pack into assigned dressing room spaces, often sharing them with other studios. Sometimes, the event is so packed there's not enough dressing space.

Once, this happened to us, and our dancers were directed to some pop-up pipe and drape in the downstairs lobby of the venue. Our parents were outraged that they were paying the same price as the other dancers but were not receiving the same experience. At the time, the complaints seemed frivolous in comparison to all of the other concerns, but in retrospect, their argument is completely valid.

On all accounts, decorum in the competitive dance space is an afterthought, which is particularly surprising when you remember the overall price point of the experience. If you consider how it feels to attend a show versus how it feels to attend a dance competition, the two environments are opposites.

## INFLEXIBILITY

Nothing about the competitive dance sphere encourages flexibility. If a conflict arises and someone must miss a rehearsal or event, it impacts the entire group. The group becomes upset because their child's ability to shine is now impacted by someone they now perceive as not caring about the overall well-being of the group.

The reason for the miss doesn't matter: illness, funeral, opportunity, school. I've dealt with every excuse and reason imaginable, and unfortunately, it was rare for the group's response to be rooted in compassion or understanding.

This led to us creating a strict policy regarding attendance, which was met with even more discontent. We were in a lose-lose position.

People want to do what they want on their own terms.

They may not want to travel six times a semester.

They may not want to use their vacation budget for a ten-day, national convention/competition.

As I gained wisdom and age, I began to understand their perspective.

When I started respecting myself and my personal time, it all made sense.

The lack of adaptability and flexibility in the competitive sphere was a barrier to reaching the fullest potential of my brand and my business, and in the process, it was creating frustration upon frustration for all involved.

## THE CONSIDERATION OF FAMILY VALUES

Client values and the family construct is important to consider. Does the competitive sphere support the needs of the current American family? With multiple children, multi-income households, and a myriad of demands, is this industry an asset or a hindrance to building quality, engaging family time?

During our days in the competitive sphere, I was a work-horse. I vacationed for work and bookended my work weeks with working weekends. My inner circle eventually brought it to my attention that my work habits were crazy and unsustainable.

This change of pace forced me to look beyond my own personal view.

The Allen Family perfectly summarized the struggle of finding balance, catering to different needs, and accommodating the perceived societal standard of "advancement":

> "As parents of young children, we discussed at length the idea of our kids not dictating our schedules as parents and the desire to create family values. One of the values important to us was spending family time together and allowing our kids to have time for free play. Three kids later, these ideas and values are very difficult to maintain. The culture around us doesn't give many options.

When you begin an extracurricular activity at a young age, it's not long before the conversation shifts to 'let us tell you about our competitive team' or 'it's just one more practice a week and one more game.' Before long, a child is eight years old, practicing four to five nights a week, traveling every other weekend just to be on the lowest-level competition team.

The idea of a family meal quickly becomes a drive-thru dinner and eating in the car together going to the next activity. Free time dissipates as practices and homework increase. And this is all happening for an eight-year-old. Imagine the pressure for families as kids get older. It's hard to not think you're doing something wrong if you say no."

With this perspective, it is easy to see the immense pressure we put on ourselves to conform and excel because "it's the thing to do," even when it is contrary to our inclination and purpose. I was guilty of it.

I also had a gut feeling that a lot of people might breathe a sigh of relief if the weight and expectation was released from our programming and replaced with something more meaningful, cost-efficient, and flexible.

## BAD FOR BUSINESS

In my experience, if a student won, they were too good for our program.

If a student lost, we were not providing adequate training.

I no longer felt comfortable with my qualitative rating being tied to a deregulated industry with no consistency or predictability. I knew the value of the technique and training I had to offer, and I did not want it being questioned because of an industry with a multitude of visible and arguable flaws.

My clients assumed I was making a considerable profit on the competitive program (as sensible business models would). I was not. Our team was nicely sized, but it was not large enough to turn a profit. I saw the invoices coming in and going out. It's a lot of money. I understood the perception, even if it was inaccurate for our model.

Beyond that, I couldn't shake the acknowledgment of the amount of resources our competitive team demanded—instructionally and administratively. There was an emotional toll that was exhausting and draining. The team represented only 10 percent of our studio population, yet it consumed a much higher percentage in time and financial resources.

Clients were not recruited and retained because of our competitive division. They stayed because they believed in our mission and our overall programming. I feared other areas of our programming were not receiving the attention they deserved because of the cumbersome amount of time and energy competitions were demanding.

I was right, and as soon as I recognized the potential for growth and development in other areas of our business, the game changed.

## THE BIG BUCKS

The competitive dance industry costs consumers (the dance studio clients) a lot of money: travel, hotels, entry fees, costumes, etc. Much of the fees are laundered through the dance studios, as the competitions only accept payments from the studio owner to "minimize" the chance of unethical competition.

The competitive dance industry has deep pockets.

In the dance studio industry, they are the "big business" and have their hand in almost everything.

They sponsor magazine ads in our industry publications, produce the largest educational events in the industry, are involved with dance studio consulting agencies, and offer kickback trips to their most valuable clientele.

The dance competition Showstopper publishes a full glossy magazine self-promoted as "The #1 Teen Dance Magazine." The Spring 2020 edition has Taylor Swift on the cover, and, intermixed with typical teen magazine features such as quizzes and fashion, are propaganda-style pieces like "7

Dancers on Their Journey to Winning the Iconic, Coveted Crystal Trophy" or "View From The Top: A Quick Look at Our 2019 National Finals Winners."[11]

For the Break the Floor Exclusive VIP Studio Owner Retreat in 2019, studio owners plus one guest were invited on a six-day, five-night stay at the W Paris Opera from December 10 to December 15, 2019, in Paris, France. To qualify for the trip, the studio had to spend $22,500 or more in fees (collectively) for Break the Floor events in the 2018–2019 competitive season.[12]

While the studio owners and guest were responsible for airfare and incidentals, the competition covered hotel rooms, a welcome cocktail party, tickets to the Moulin Rouge, dinner at Le Refuge Des Fondus (where they touted you can drink wine out of baby bottles), French wine tasting, and a cruise on the Seine River.

The "VIP Guest List" listed more than three hundred studios as eligible to attend.

The studios that participate in a big way have major incentive to continue. The mid- to smaller-size studios continue

11   *Showstopper Magazine*, Spring 2020.

12   "Break the Floor: Exclusive VIP Studio Owner Retreat, Paris, France, December 10th-15th, 2019, W Paris Opera," accessed December 5, 2019, breakthefloor.com.

to compete because they feel there are no alternative options.

**You will not hear many counterarguments for the dance competition industry in the secular dance space, because it is financially dominated by the competitive market.**

It is a big, big bear. Because of deregulation, there's no official data or statistics. When subsets of the industry try to formalize, they tend to spiral out of control or dissolve. That's what happened to the Federation of Dance Competitions. There's no regulation, no tracking, no accountability.

A *New York Times* piece offered that 52,000 children attended the Showstopper competition in 2016.[13] That represents one competition out of hundreds that exist. Thousands of studios across the United States participate in dance competitions each year.

The numbers we can track are staggering, and that's why this conversation is a necessity.

Big impact is happening.

---

13   Lizzie Feidelson, "Inside the High Drama World of Youth Competition Dance," *New York Times*, December 21, 2017, https://www.nytimes.com/2017/12/21/magazine/inside-the-high-drama-world-of-youth-competition-dance.html.

Is it the type of impact we want to see as we look toward a strong, powerful, and creative future in dance education?

Ultimately, as I weighed my pros and cons, I realized the negative actualities, possibilities, and perceptions within this industry were overwhelmingly counterproductive to facilitating a program that empowered and inspired every child. That had always been my goal, and as I leaned into the feedback and research, I recognized we had veered entirely off track.

Knowledge is power when we use it. Activation is key.

*Chapter 4*

# MAKE THE MOVES

Life is busy, and adulting is hard. We all have lists of things we hope to accomplish. I fear that so many people leave their lists of hopes and dreams collecting cobwebs in a deserted corner.

Don't let this happen to you!

With passion as the foundation and the pros/cons as the launch point, hold yourself accountable for making some major moves. Grab an accountability buddy, find sources of inspiration, and get to work. Change is usually inconvenient, but it is so worth it to elevate your offerings to this world and to your life.

For me, once the "ick factor" of something is identified, everything wrong is exacerbated. It happened with our run in the competitive dance industry, and it has happened in other areas of my life. Going down the rabbit hole is tough, but in that darkness is enlightenment.

With the looming shift out of the competitive dance industry, there were months where I felt so stressed about the knowledge I had versus the action I was delaying. My therapist tells me now that avoidance is simply rescheduling conflict, and boy, was I a master of rescheduling it. I'd break out in hives in Target. I'd feel anxious opening the studio email. I'd sit in the parking lot and shed a few tears. When the phone would ring, I'd feel a jolt of stress shoot through my body. I'd try to busy myself with as many things as possible to distract myself from the continued chaos. I would bend over backward to please everyone but myself.

One of the most frustrating parts of this journey was how easy it was to lose sight of rational perspective. The issues created as a by-product of the competitive dance industry can feel so big. Yet, they're solvable problems very much within our control. Within the isolated bubble of the dance competition industry, routine adjudication and placement and other trivial things feels so grandiose. In the real world and on a scale of major, impacting life events, it just doesn't matter. It's crazy how we can be pulled into these trivial conflicts.

While attending one competitive event, I found out one of

our five-year-old students passed away. That's a real-life issue, and my heart sank to the depths of my stomach. I felt nauseous as I drove home that day.

The child joined our programming when he was three years old. He was so joyful and loved to dance. When his cancer recurred, his mother requested private lessons since they likely would not have a mother/son first dance together at a wedding. They chose "Tomorrow" from the musical *Annie* as their song, and even though we never finished the routine, we captured rehearsal footage that is the penultimate representation of the power of the performing arts.

As I attended the child's funeral, I was also fielding emails questioning adjudications and why certain routines were not scoring higher than they were at the weekend's competition. I felt gutted in dividing my attention between a family experiencing insufferable, real loss and entertaining questions about seemingly irrelevant, trivial issues involving competitive dance.

You cannot direct how or why people place value on certain things or situations, or how they lose sight of the things that really matter. It can certainly confuse you and prompt a lot of thought and conversation, but most importantly, it affirms the rightness in making moves.

Complacency enables the status quo.

This juxtaposition of values and meaning was an awakening for me. I had one foot out the competitive industry door when one of my long-term (and still with me) studio moms sent a list of very rational observations about her first-time experience at a convention.

I was exhausted and did not want to hear it, but I needed to hear it. The challenges from rational, pragmatic perspectives were my lifeline at a time when I was desperate for guidance.

Points included:

- Praise for the convention instructors, specifically noting how they applied technical skills to life skills.
- Concern about the daytime Friday scheduling, explaining that she prefers not to interrupt her child's education with extracurricular activities
- Concern that the convention and hotel were not prepared for the crowd
- The security guards had several inappropriate altercations with parents, including physical interactions and profane language.
- The closing awards ceremony was chaotic.
- The photo sales booth was inefficient and poorly organized.
- Her daughter did not understand how the judging works and how subjective it can be.

I read it, soaked in the information, and realized her observations were a direct reflection of my own thoughts. I wrote a thoughtful response addressing what I could and lamenting on mutually agreeable flaws and concerns.

Her response was appreciative and casual, but it deeply resonated with me.

> "I'm trying to practice what I talk to the kids about all the time—using my voice for things I care about. We appreciate what you do for our kids and the studio. Thanks!"

The phrase that resonated with me was:

**"I'm trying to practice what I talk to the kids about all the time—using my voice for the things I care about."**

That was the wake-up call my apathy needed.

What did I care about?

It wasn't dance competitions.

And it wasn't the culture they were creating at my studio.

When circumstances are in your control, there is no honor in playing the victim. I knew it was go time. I was ready to make the moves! I wanted to cultivate meaningful and unique experiences that created community at an affordable price point and return on investment. I wanted to spread love for the performing arts, and I wanted to do it in a way that was empowering and inspiring to others.

I wanted to create a program that I could be excited and proud for my child to be a part of. Long-term legacy was on my mind. What could I create that aligned with my values and experiences that could exist and thrive long after I'm gone?

That's what I cared about.

That's what I was going to do.

*"She remembered who she was and the game changed."*
—LALAH DELIA

By the time I decided to roll out the change, I'd sat on the notion and possibility for years. It was time to organize, eliminate distraction, and go all in to see if I could innovate and redirect our path, which had strayed slightly off course. Sometimes, the inspiration we need to prompt our change is right in front of us.

Growing up, I always enjoyed theatre. Well, I take that back. I was terrified when I auditioned to be a child of Siam in *The King and I* in third grade at Actors Coming Together in

Greeneville, Tennessee. I wasn't cast in that show, but once I was eventually cast in a production (*Babes in Toyland* at the Little Theatre of Greeneville), I found a sense of belonging which carried through to my college degree.

When the studio first opened, I had to forgo my participation in theatre, as I was fully focused on the studio. I maintained my role as an enthusiastic audience member and looked forward to the day when I could participate again. I was especially excited to transition my skills as a performer to the creative teams. Behind the scenes is where I shine.

Amid the business's turmoil, the opportunity presented itself to rediscover my love for the stage as a choreographer and director. These roles became my catharsis and inspiration during a very challenging period for my business. In six years, I worked on thirty-six productions, ranging from high school to community to children's theatre to regional theatre to sensory-aware performances.

Each experience was an opportunity:

- To be reminded about the true power of performance without the pursuit of accolades
- To experience the feeling that community performance can generate when it is appropriately structured
- To build relationships with people from different backgrounds that share a common love for performing arts

- To achieve a goal that is rooted in the trifecta of personal progress, team accomplishment, and audience enjoyment
- To share the experience of artistic creation and storytelling between performer and audience member

Don't get me wrong—the theatre world isn't a drama-free utopia. Yet, even with the occasional challenges, I learned a lot about my strengths, weaknesses, and how to be a committed, semi-fearless leader. I learned more about myself and what I wanted for my life and my legacy. I found confidence in making tough decisions for the betterment of the whole. I received good theatre reviews and not-so-great theatre reviews, which helped me regain confidence in my work that was not reliant on external perceptions and opinions. "Up or out" became my motto, and I decided I was going UP in all areas of my life.

The experiences in theatre neutralized my negative experiences in the competitive dance industry and graced me with the opportunity to make some radical corrections in my businesses. Dance and theatre are synergetic, yet different. Inspiration often emerges in the unlikeliest of places, and I felt confident I could perfectly blend the best of the two into our programming.

## GETTING DOWN TO BUSINESS

When change feels SO right, it is almost burdensome to have to wait for it. I was ready to delve into molding a program that offered quality training with an exceptional return on investment. And I wanted it done yesterday.

Once the change process is activated, you may:

- Feel grief and/or gratitude for different elements of the experiences
- Identify lessons learned
- Second-guess the transformation
- Have your beliefs questioned and challenged

Embrace and recognize every feeling and emotion because it is critical and necessary for surviving the next phase of your journey. Change is hard and inconvenient. Prepare for that now.

When your change aligns with your core values, mission, and legacy, the other side of the transformation will be more than worth it. You can do it!

# Chapter 5

# PREPARE FOR
# THE STORM

On my high school notebook, I had the following quote:

*"I am not afraid of storms, for I am learning how to sail my ship."*

—LOUISA MAY ALCOTT

When change, conflict, or transition is in front of us, we become paralyzed to facing reality because we are so fearful of response, reputation, and perception. We prepare for blizzards, flat tires, and the first day of school, but societally, we neglect to psychologically prepare for major life changes and emotional events.

When I tell people about leaving the competitive dance industry, the number-one question I receive is:

**Weren't you afraid of what others would think?**

Yes. Absolutely.

I was terrified. I was afraid of losing clients. I was afraid of losing staff.

(All of which happened.)

I was afraid of losing my dream.

(That didn't happen.)

I was also afraid of losing my credibility, something I worked tirelessly to build.

In addition to the studios, I had a relatively successful blog and seminar series, *The Dance Exec*, which operated from 2013 to 2016. *The Dance Exec* offered a free online resource series to dance educators as well as seminar events in Charlotte and Raleigh, North Carolina, and New York City.

I loved connecting with educators and tapped into so much information about the national and global dance scene. I saw hopes, dreams, deficiencies, passion, and potential, but most of all, I saw people who cared deeply about their art and educating others.

Conversations about the competition industry were a large part of the online resource series. On the blog, I wrote a prolific seventy-nine pieces categorized as devoted to the competitive dance industry. When I revisited the content series, the timeline and growing intensity of my frustration and disdain are so evident. There's a post from July 1, 2015, "What Happens When They Take Away the Trophy?" that basically foreshadows the entire premise of this book.

It's crazy how something can be happening in our lives and we don't even realize it until it's whacking us over the head with a mallet, *Looney Tunes*-style.

I reached a point where I felt unmotivated to continue offering wisdom and advice because I felt fraudulent and hypocritical. For four years, I published content four days a week. I knew it was time to put the pen down to focus on action instead of advice. I sold the content of the blog to TutuTix, a dance-oriented ticketing company I respect and admire. I knew it would live on in perpetuity without requiring my daily attention.

In managing the guilt-laden feelings of walking away from the competitive dance industry, I had to abandon the notion that my reputation of success was affiliated with this micro-piece of the larger dance industry. I wrestled with the perception that our studio's brand and identity was established because of our participation in competitions. Several of my network, connections, and friends were largely fostered through the competitive dance scene. Would I be ostracized? Would our branding be devalued because of this shift?

There's a point where the commitment to the cause is greater than the fear of criticism.

I reached that point.

How do you walk away from something without looking like a failure?

1. Strategically prepare.
2. Confidently communicate.
3. Passionately believe in the outcome.

## STRATEGICALLY PREPARE

During strategic preparations, it is important to identify your ideal outcome with a major transition or change.

For my journey, I needed to:

1. Make sure the root of the problem was a by-product of the culture perpetuated within the competitive dance industry and not some other type of influence or source.
2. Research and activate ways I could replace the positive

components of the competitive dance industry so that I could still offer reputable training for our dancers interested in pursuing dance/performing-arts education at a more intense level.

3. Inform my staff and leadership about the change. Buy-in from your immediate support structure is important. For the people who do not buy-in, it is important to be okay with parting ways. You cannot force your views on others.

For the outcome, I wanted to create a program that was a stronger, more meaningful return on investment than the competitive dance scene. If this was a successful transition, I was confident we could boost our overall enrollment, mission, and impact.

## CONFIDENTLY COMMUNICATE

People are programmed to resist change. Human instinct tends to lean into the fear of the unknown versus embracing the excitement of possibility.

That's an important piece to consider when you are preparing to communicate your change. While you've been observing, preparing, and activating strategy, the other party has continued to subscribe to the status quo.

The news will be unsettling and may evoke feelings of misunderstanding, distrust, or a wrongful attack. If possible, change can be easier to understand if there's a middle ground, an option that bridges the former state to the new state.

Here are five strategies to use when communicating this type of information:

1. Determine the appropriate medium. In determining the appropriate medium, ask yourself how the information will best be received. Is it an in-person conversation, or is it better suited for a written format? What are the risks relating to miscommunication or misperception?
2. Practice. Envision and practice every scenario imaginable. I always start with "What's the worst that could happen?" From there, I practice and strategize every imaginable possibility. For this exercise, let your creativity run wild. Mentally prepare for the worst and hope for the best.
3. Educate. Knowledge is power. Do your backend research, so you can be prepared for questions, suggestions, thoughts, and feedback. Keep your tone even and avoid condescension, even if you feel you have been wronged. Blame is not a productive use of energy.
4. Listen. The other party will likely want to be heard. If the conversation is being respectfully managed, listen. Even if we do not agree with counterarguments or opinions, if we listen, we gain a deeper understanding of the

human condition through empathy. This helps us make better decisions and choices in the future.

5.  Be steadfast. If you are about to go through a pivot or a change, this is not the time to waver on your beliefs or actions. Be strong, confident, and committed. Frame your narrative with hope, excitement, and enthusiasm. To create a movement and gain followers, you must be confident in your strategy and execution.

When we transitioned out of the competitive dance industry, we decided to individually meet with every family who was participating in the competitive component. As much as I dreaded the conversations, I knew they were necessary. The clients had been a part of my program for multiple years, and I felt like they deserved to hear about the transition directly from me, even though I knew many would respond with resistance and/or may feel disappointment toward my leadership choices. Conversations about change are tough!

On a sunny May afternoon, we pulled a table out in the back-studio room and prepared for hours of conversation. I was anxious and terrified. We had put so much time and consideration into our new concept that I hoped people would respect it, even if they didn't subscribe to it.

The feedback was varied. Most people predicted a change was coming, and most of our clients used it as a cordial way to exit our competitive program and studio without any further extreme levels of negativity, conflict, or toxicity. During one meeting, a mom said: "This program seems much truer to what you've always said you represent." That stayed with me, and for the first time in a long time, I felt like I was using my voice for the right reasons.

*"There is only one way to avoid criticism: do nothing, say nothing, be nothing."*

—ARISTOTLE

Even if the initial receiving parties of change are pleasant and respectful during in-person interactions, it does not mean the respect will continue. When people react, it reflects their own experiences, beliefs, and values.

People may be quick to jump to an overly defensive stance regarding their continued participation in something you are choosing to leave. It's important to mentally prepare for assumptions people might project toward your positioning:

- She wasn't successful enough.
- Her program wasn't big enough.
- Her best students left her.
- Her best staff left the program.
- Her choreography wasn't good enough.
- She wouldn't listen to us.
- Our costumes weren't fancy enough.

- She's too conservative in her costuming and choreography.
- She didn't hire enough outside choreographers.
- She didn't lead a full barre before the dancers went on stage.
- She didn't style my French twist.
- She didn't stand in the lobby of the studio.
- She wouldn't walk to the studio in the snow for my child's private lesson.
- She didn't care enough about winning.

Most of these statements were actually said during and immediately after our change—some were true, some were false, some were heightened and exaggerated. Some will probably resurface with the publication of this book.

Even though I attempted to prepare for this type of negativity on the back end, the power of critical words can be intense. Keep in mind: criticism is only as powerful as the energy we give it. It is so hard to separate from it, but it is one of the greatest acts of self-kindness and self-care.

When you are experiencing change, go ahead and own the counternarrative so you can be prepared to stand above it. And even when things are said that aren't true, take a moment to identify the root of the perception. There's a solid chance the behavior isn't about you, and instead, it is about the other person's experience. Most importantly, let your actions stand alongside your words.

The first time you create controversy is the most difficult. When you become the "bad person," it's likely because you took the initiative to stand for something that conflicted with someone else's core perception or values. You created a conversation, which most people never have the confidence or tenacity to do.

I care about people and consider myself a unifier, but I have made radical moves over the years, I have ruffled some feathers along the way:

- When I launched *The Dance Exec*, I naively sent out a press release to every contact I could find, including the dance industry's major media outlets. One of the companies had an editor who "replied all" (I do not think she meant to include me on the email) with the following message: "Wow, give this woman an award for self-promotion."
- When I realized a community theatre was not operating to the technical standards required to produce consistent, quality performances to support their talented base of volunteer performers, I sent a professional letter resigning from any future work at that particular location. I was ostracized for that move, but I had to make it; otherwise, I would enable the cycle of technical inadequacy.

- In business, there is always a sprinkling of negative online reviews. They are hurtful and generally reflect a culture clash between the client expectations and the program operations. Most of the time, the reviewer does not directly reach out to us and will not respond to our follow-ups. That's frustrating. One of my friends taught me years ago that "the internet is a platform for belligerence," and since hearing that, I try to consciously spread more positivity than negativity online. I encourage you to do the same!

With purpose-driven work, there's a stronger mental capacity for managing the chaos. As a leader and innovator, it is important to know your triggers, what you will and will not stand for, and who you truly are as a person and what you represent. There's nothing wrong with self-advocacy, and with experience, you'll gain wisdom regarding what's wrong, what's right, and what requires distance.

When you're in the storm, remember:

- Conflict leads to innovation.
- Innovation creates change.
- Change brings opportunity.
- All will be met with varying levels of resistance.

In our movement, the first step was to rebrand the name of the program to match its mission. Our competition team was called the Stage Door Elite, which was an elementary lesson in the importance of naming and branding. With *Elite* in the name, it made it more accessible for people to approach their participation with "elite" attitudes.

I wanted a purposeful title that accurately represented our mission and direction.

We landed on calling the new program the Intensive Training Program.

Drastic changes were happening. If they happened all at once, it would be overwhelming to participants. There's a threshold for change acceptance, and the tipping point of too much change can be met with extreme reactions.

We opted to offer clients a transition period for our first year "out" of the competitive dance industry. We offered a dual-track intensive experience: (a) the primary Intensive Training Program and (b) the Competitive Focus Experience, an add-on supplement that would allow students to compete in solos or duos on their own with assistance, but not with direct endorsement from the studio. While that may sound hypocritical, it was strategically designed, and it was the right avenue to take within the circumstances. We wanted to build more bridges than we burned.

Four words would serve as the core value pillars of the Intensive Training Program:

1. Technique
2. Performance
3. Community
4. Character

Everything in the program would need to reference back to one of these words.

Our first official season of our new program was 2015–2016. The students would continue taking their classes in an inclusive way (as it had always been), and we would offer an Intensive Training Program Focus Session on Wednesday evenings for the students to set their choreography and work on their community and character components.

This is the announcement our clients received as we started outwardly marketing the new program:

> "In seven years, Stage Door Dance Productions has established itself as a premier leader in dance education on a local and national level. We believe that this success stems from our solid training and quality service, along with our underlying and ultimate belief in the strength of our organization. As the dance industry evolves, we must also re-evaluate our

purpose and determine the methods required to best serve our students.

The competitive dance industry is moving towards an extremely competitive environment that lacks focus, direction, standardization, and regulation. While competitive experience is one way to improve the performer, relying solely on dance competitions to further dance education is not an effective means to training the higher quality level of dancers and performers that our studio aspires to train. Thus, the competitive component of the Intensive Training Program will be transitioning to a supplementary element of the program that will eventually become nonexistent.

The Intensive Training Program is significantly redesigned for the upcoming Dance Season, will shift the focus off of the competitive aspect, and will ultimately focus on four pillars of personal growth development: technique, performance, community, and character.

We understand that being a part of this program is a significant investment of time, finances, and commitment, and we have spent a considerable amount of time determining options that will result in the best return on investment for your dancer(s). We understand that our newly designed program may not work for every dancer and we encourage you to consider our program ONLY if our infrastructure works for you.

The goal of the Stage Door Dance Intensive Training Program is to encourage dancers to achieve their highest potential by providing the highest level of technical and stylistic dance training. To accomplish this goal in a positive manner, we will redirect the focus of parents, students, and teachers to the accomplishments achieved through the learning experience.

Long-term, it is most beneficial for our dancers to receive a solid technical foundation. This will prepare dancers to be adaptable to various styles and methods of instruction while remaining versatile and humble. This is also more aligned with the professional dance industry.

The goals of the Intensive Training Program are as follows:

1. Provide strong technical and performance training in a variety of dance styles.

2. Create a flexible environment that will accommodate the exploration of additional interests (auditioning and participating in theatrical performances, participating in school/extracurricular activities, training in music/acting/voice, etc.).

3. Explore opportunities that focus on community and character, encouraging our dancers' success on and offstage.

The Stage Door Dance Intensive Training Program recognizes that winning does not come in the shape of a trophy or medal. Rather, it is being able to recognize the journey we choose to live and the ability and awareness to be grateful for it.

As we moved into the new era, we also evaluated how we could infuse more brand consistency into the other elements of our program.

The beginning steps included:

- Eliminating competitive dialogue from our studio vocabulary. The focus fully shifted to inclusivity of all. All our dancers are trained with relative difficulty, teaching them in an appropriate way for their educational style.
- If a student opted to participate in the Intensive Training Program, the dialogue was presented as "heightened training opportunities."
- Eliminating person-to-person comparative language and focusing on positive individual feedback, progress, and encouragement.
- Removing the presumption of leveled placement, we redesigned our placement process to cohorts. The cohorts are evaluated specifically for each season and are nonnumerical since numbers are psychologically affiliated to the school grading system.
- Redeveloping our dress code to require a leotard base

with tights/shorts/leggings over the leotard (depending on the style of dance). Our rationale explains that this is for uniformity, safety, and a distraction-free dance environment.

Then, we held our breath.

With storms, there's always the calm before, the chaos during, and the cleanup of the aftermath. Nerves and anxiety swell around the unknown. Big decisions and emotional life events often have the same experience pattern. As much as we'd like for them to happen and be over, with little to no impact, that's usually not the case.

With strategic preparations, confident communication, and a passionate optimism about the other side of the change, you will persevere. And, most likely, there will even be a rainbow on the other side.

*Chapter 6*

# OWN YOUR NARRATIVE

Have you ever heard, "It's 11:11—make a wish!"? After activating the program change, I wished on anything and everything I could find. I bought healing stones, had my chakras balanced, saged the buildings, and consciously made a wish every time the clock hit 11:11.

Please, make this work.

Please, let people buy into this concept.

It felt SO right, and I wanted everyone to be as excited as I was.

They weren't—not at all.

And that's often how big decisions go. You may be so excited and ready to activate big change, but the response may not be as initially enthusiastic as you might have hoped. Stick with it. Building a movement takes time.

Eighty percent of our competitive students initially on our competitive team left to compete at other dance studios. It hurt my ego because my intention was in the right place with the program redevelopment. It was frustrating to recognize my inability to lead our entire population to this new concept. I wanted the ecosystem to heal instead of continuing to hurt. I didn't realize this at the time, but in extracting the people who were completely tied to the competitive culture, I created the first big step in the recovery process.

While I didn't get the initial buy-in I wanted, I provided an opportunity for people to leave without an extreme negative exchange. That was smart. Even some of our families who had nothing against the studio chose to leave. Other families hurt their feelings, or they were exhausted from the extreme amount of negativity. Can you imagine running a business where people are hurt or exhausted from extreme fatigue of negativity? It wasn't what I wanted, and I felt sad we had reached this point under my leadership.

Our competitive team had fifty participants in the 2014–2015 season.

Our new Intensive Training Program had thirteen participants in the 2015–2016 season.

If you build it, they will come...

Or, at least, that is the hope.

One misconception about implementing radical change is that you will immediately see results.

Sadly, that's not the case. The moments of transformation are quiet, somewhat isolated, and lonely. You may question your choice and wonder if what you abandoned will be worth what's coming. Nobody is standing next to you popping champagne with a confetti cannon and parading around singing your praises and calling you a game changer. In fact, people aren't even really talking to you because people fear change. They'll call you crazy before they jump on board.

Building a movement takes time. If something feels ethically irresponsible, you cannot refute the truth or the facts in order to solely protect your bottom line. Life is a series of experiments.

If you aren't moving, you're standing still.

During the early days of the new program, there were signs that we were on the right track.

Our overall enrollment was increasing, and there was space to breathe. The cloud of intensity was lifting.

A couple of years into the new program, I had lunch with my friend Sandy. I was feeling kind of down on myself and frustrated that we were not leveraging the traction and excitement we initially hoped. With tears in my eyes, I looked at her and said, "There are some days where I just don't know—" Midsentence, she stopped me. She looked me in the eye and matter-of-factly said, "You have always been about so much more than the average dance studio..."

It was an honest exchange. She genuinely meant what she said, and it lifted my spirits.

There are moments when we all need that type of real, in-your-face motivational exchange, and I try to be diligent in giving as much as I receive. Empowerment fuels the world and pushes us to our potential.

As the day continued, I kept thinking about the words "Stage Door" and "more."

My mind flashed back.

Before the studio opened, it was working under the name "Studio C."

In November 2008, I was in New York City seeing a binge of Broadway shows. As I passed the stage doors on Broadway, I thought about everything the stage door represents: accomplishment, hard work, storytelling, performance, connection, community, and focus. At that moment, amid the magic of the Great White Way, I knew the studio was meant to be called Stage Door Dance Productions.

With the "more" component, I am obsessed with leveling up. Let's not stop with what is in front of us; let's not stop with what's easy. Let's be the best version of a dance studio we can imagine. Let's be the best version of a children's extracurricular program we can imagine. Let's learn so much about business inside and out that we make smart, calculated, strategic decisions, so that we can do anything we imagine.

Let's:

Be

More

At

Stage

Door.

The motto/hashtag was born, and we use it extensively. It guides our work, keeps us on track, sets boundaries, and represents a heightened level of accountability for the business and the brand.

The Be More mentality is a universal guiding principle that expands far beyond the studio.

It works for personal and professional goals and captures the essence of a favorite African proverb:

> Every morning in Africa, a gazelle wakes up. It knows it must move faster than the lion or it will not survive. Every morning a lion wakes up and it knows it must move faster than the slowest gazelle or it will starve. It doesn't matter if you are the lion or the gazelle, when the sun comes up, you better be moving.

Move the Needle. Ignite the Change. Make it Better.

Intention is powerful. The thought that goes into something directly translates to the output. Meaning and messaging that is purposeful is so much stronger than a hollow action, and that's what builds strong brands. I did not think about this enough in our early days; now, I make sure our intentions and branding are always consistently aligned.

Honesty, transparency, vulnerability, and self-awareness

are all key in the messaging you use to build buy-in and a brand. It may take time and missteps, and that's okay. Once you reach a truly purposeful message, vision, and brand, the rest will fall into place.

*Chapter 7*

# LEVEL UP

If you've made it to the point of committing to a major change or rebrand, you have endless opportunities ahead. How will you use this opportunity to correct professional or personal weaknesses while also leveling up and exceeding expectations? In curating our program, I knew I wanted to create something revolutionary for our dancers.

In the period immediately prior to our rebranding, my creativity was struggling. I was walking through the motions, but my brain wasn't firing ideas at its typical pace. Everything felt hazy. Once there was a bit of stability, my creativity started returning because my brain had the space to dream and play.

While the bulk of my work is rooted in the performing arts, the need for creativity is universally applicable in any business model. Creativity is required for marketing, problem-solving, program development, and corporate vision. It's also required for a happy and fulfilled life. Acknowledging what fuels and hinders your creativity is important in setting a productive pace for your business's success.

Creative energy is a lot like Tinkerbell. When you are happy, grounded, fulfilled, supported, and rested, your creativity overflows and shines your bright light. When you are stressed, anxious, fearful, and lack support, your creative energy diminishes, and your bright light dwindles.

For four years, between 2014 and 2018, I choreographed Ira David Wood III's *A Christmas Carol*, a celebrated holiday show tradition in Raleigh, North Carolina.

In the show's finale, a chorus of children sing the following line:

*"Pretty dreams don't ever die; they just wait for you and I..."*

Year after year, I would pause at the power of this lyric. I felt like it was speaking directly to me.

The lyric affirmed my belief that the dance studio's greatest potential for success and impact lay in what I envisioned, dreamed about, and loved as a child: the ability to connect, communicate, and heal through the dance education experience.

For our new program, performance was the baseline, but what would make the Intensive Training Program a next-level experience?

Four factors guided the way:

1. Performance
2. Service
3. Experience
4. Empowerment

## PERFORMANCE

As a child, I could hardly sleep the night before my dance recital. I was so excited and lived for opportunities to perform. How could we capture that level of magic in our students' training?

The performance component is a necessity for the performing arts. Students crave this level of structure and discipline to recognize and respect the goal-oriented process of building and curating a performance. This is an introduction to project management at its finest!

With our new program, how could we educate about the

importance of the performance process while also discovering new and creative ways to present our repertoire of routines?

Through the process of performance, students gain:

- Self-esteem
- Self-assurance
- Self-confidence

The experience prepares students for:

- Performing arts opportunities
- In-school presentations
- Improved socialization
- Targeted goal achievement

The practice/rehearsal process encourages:

- Retention skills
- Responsibility and accountability
- Self-discipline
- Time management
- Goal setting and achievement
- Adaptability and resilience
- Collaborative team planning and execution

People assume the dance recital model is comparably

exploitative to the competitive dance industry, and that is false. In our year-end recital, we avoid elaborate stage makeup designs, inappropriate songs, and revealing costumes. They're not a part of our culture. In every aspect, we believe that children should be children, and our recital is heralded as the celebratory capstone to the main performance season.

While the recital is wonderful, it would not suffice as the only performance component for our Intensive Training Program experience. From the get-go, I started emailing every festival, venue, and contact I could find. I wanted to duplicate the performance experience as much as possible to allow our students the most practical performance experience available in our area.

From arts festivals to the children's museum to the Golden Years Proms to parades along the East Coast, we have performed in nearly every scenario imaginable. One of the best parts? It duplicates the performance element of the dance competition experience in a more entertainment industry-oriented setting for zero cost.

I remember the first time we went to the veterans' hospital in Durham to perform. Several of our students were shocked at the patients' conditions: some veterans were in wheelchairs; some were amputees. They were a receptive, gracious, and enthusiastic audience. The veterans enjoyed every second of the performance, and our students gained a heightened sense of awareness about the world around them.

I recognized we have so much work to do in building local and global awareness in our students. I want our students to understand the scope of the power of their art. While it can serve their talents, it can also positively impact the world and cultivate their confidence and leadership, on and off the stage. The giving of the art is equal to the receiving of the talent. Our audience options were endless because dance is a universal language—it transcends age, language, and circumstance. This notion was important and pivotal in the uniqueness of our reinvention.

## SERVICE

My heart has always been service-oriented—helping others has always felt very natural. Extending that philosophy into the studio made perfect sense. When we first transitioned to the Intensive Training Program, we started with small service projects such as penny wars for the animal shelter and donation drives.

The intent of our service component was always in the right place, but our greatest opportunity was discovered when one of my staff members, Amy, pulled me aside. Amy and I have been friends for a very long time and her daughter was my first student in our very first summer camp. Five years later, I opened our second location when Amy agreed to sign on as the director. She lived through the competition days, and on a Friday morning around 5:00 a.m. at a competitive event in Charlotte, we deliriously looked at each other and mutually agreed the time was right to exit.

In 2016, Amy was serving on the board for a locally founded nonprofit, Global H2O. The organization was looking for groups to host fundraisers to raise $7,500 to fund clean water wells in Uganda. She mentioned this to me as a potential opportunity for our new Intensive Training Program. I thought about the idea, felt a little overwhelmed by it, and then decided to do it. I wanted to do it in the best way we knew how: by putting on a show. After all, the best things tend to happen when we stretch ourselves outside of our comfort zone doing what we know best.

When I first announced the plan to our team, one of our former staff members told me to mentally prepare myself to write a check out of my savings account because I was going to embarrass myself with a big, fat failure. Ouch. I've never shied away from a challenge, and in my heart, I knew we could do this. One morning, while drinking out of my Kate Spade coffee mug, I looked at the bottom where it colorfully says, "Make a Splash!" We had a name for the show and were ready to rock.

A small theatre donated their space, and I recruited a couple of community friends to serve as guest artists. My team went all in, and like we always do, we did it. It was a humble start, but it was the beginning of something so exciting.

During the fundraising journey, I remember reading some Global H2O statistics, including a statement that said one child dies every seventeen seconds from lack of access to safe water and basic sanitation. When we were discussing philanthropy with our students, we made the metric relatable: in the length of the benefit show's opening number, six children will die. That's harrowing, powerful stuff. And now, not only were we using our art for a global purpose, we were instilling the power of children helping other children.

There wasn't a trophy at the end of the journey. There was something much more rewarding. We used our art to create community to ignite lasting global impact. Someone might be living a little bit easier because we took the time to dance for a cause that serves others beyond ourselves. That's something I can celebrate.

We raised $7,500 and funded a clean water well in Uganda. When Amy visited Uganda to oversee the installation and deliver tutus to children in the villages, we all felt like a small part of a much bigger need within a global scale. My heart nearly exploded. That's impact, and that is where the arts have the power to gain their fullest momentum and potential.

The chaos and stress of the past led us to the opportunity of our future, which is how we developed the yearly capstone piece of the Intensive Training Program: the Peer-to-Peer Philanthropic Initiative. Within the Peer-to-Peer Philanthropic Initiative, we are always seeking initiatives that will resonate with our dancers, families, and communities. We purposely choose local organizations with reachable and relatable people. The stories we support are the stories we experience.

In 2018, we were able to celebrate the memory of the five-year-old student we lost during the competitive weekend I referenced earlier. This show was called "A Concert for the Kids." We raised money for the Me Fine Foundation, a local nonprofit that provides emotional and financial support to families undergoing cancer treatment at local hospitals. We also announced a scholarship to celebrate the life of this student, the Denny Dances Scholarship, an annual scholarship designed to cover tuition expenses for a male student for one full dance season.

When we first announced the scholarship, it was powerful to see Denny's ten family members sitting in the front row and sharing in the moment. It was a palpable example of community and an amazing way to affirm Denny's legacy and spirit at our studio, experience grief and healing, and perpetuate the joy and excitement of dance to other male students.

Max Allen received the scholarship in 2019, and his mother, Jamie, eloquently describes the impact of the scholarship for her son and her family:

> "In an environment that is so heavily female-centric, the Denny Dances Scholarship became a gift to empower male dancers in the community. **It also empowers us to spread the story of our studio and the lives that have built this place.** We are excited to be part of a studio that promotes the message that "dance is for everyone.""

A Concert for the Kids was really special because, in addition to being perfectly aligned with our peer-to-peer philanthropy, it also represented a way to highlight the stories and people who have made Stage Door Dance a really special place to be. If you listen to your community and recognize the stories that are happening around you, service opportunities are easy to find.

In 2019, Amy's son, Coco, was scheduled to graduate from the Frankie Lemmon School, a predominantly privately funded inclusive preschool for children navigating developmental delays and special needs. It is an amazing school with an exceptional staff, and Coco's ability to attend was a game changer for his educational progress.

Coco and I always had a special relationship. I remember the day he was born, and I taught him his very first year at the studio. Once he joined Frankie Lemmon, I watched him progress at a rapid pace. Raising money for this exceptionally brilliant institution was a no-brainer.

One of my proudest moments was when Coco stepped out onto the stage and rocked his own interpretive dance to "Thunder" by Imagine Dragons. His confidence in independently being on the stage was a powerful testament to his journey. The audience went wild, and once again, the stories of our studios impacted the greater good of our community.

After the 2019 show, I was feeling a touch of exhaustion. It happens to the best of us. If you are an on-the-go type, it probably hits you even harder than the average person. For me, the giving and philanthropy felt great—however, creating, navigating, and communicating our new model while cultivating the necessary growth of the businesses was taking its toll.

At the moment I thought our path might be veering away from the benefit show, I picked up a newspaper and saw an article about a place called Comfort Zone Camp, a camp for children suffering bereavement from the loss of a parent or a sibling. The power of the article stopped me in my tracks. From my past, I know how important and necessary this is for children experiencing grief. I began researching Comfort Zone Camp and was considering them as the recipient of our next benefit show.

A few days later, Amy called and said, "I know you don't share your story very often, but a student who lost her father is navigating some emotions. I mentioned the details of your story to her mom, and I think they'd really benefit from a conversation with you." I invited the student and her mother to my office, and we had a delightful interaction, sharing our stories and finding commonalities. By the end of the meeting, the sweet dancer had invited me to Chili's and Disney World. I explained that I wasn't sure that could happen, but that I knew a way we could make a difference and help others who share in our experience of childhood loss. As she walked out of my office that day, she looked back and said, "I'm so glad I'm not the only one that's lost a parent."

Right there, the mission for our 2020 benefit show was born. Never lose sight of sources of inspiration, and when you're in need of a recharge, lean into them. If you keep your eyes open, power and purpose are everywhere, and it may even draw you closer to the power of your past.

This was a huge benchmark for my personal growth. Previously, I wouldn't have felt comfortable making these connections or sharing the more vulnerable parts of my story. The beauty of presence and listening is so underrated and often deprioritized amid the daily hustle and bustle.

Discovering Comfort Zone Camp offered a complete

acknowledgment of purpose combined with passion, and I wholeheartedly knew we made the right choice and were on the right track. From that moment, I vowed to be more open, more transparent, and more vulnerable as we continued to navigate our program and all its potential.

In a world that is so busy with demands, how often are you able to support causes and organizations that are important to you? The performing arts are a form of catharsis, and when you can create, perform, and celebrate in the name of something meaningful, it makes sense. It feels right.

The community involvement piece was proving to be so successful. The root of the success was in the experience, so our next step would be to identify other impactful modes of experiential, performing arts education.

## EXPERIENCE

In affirming our "dance is for everyone" attitude, I thought about some of the projects that meant the most to me early in my teaching career:

- I created the Sightless Rhythm Tap Project at the Governor Morehead School for the Blind, a tap dance program that taught blind students basic tap dance and rhythm skills. The end of the experience featured a show.
- I wrote a dance patch for the Girls Scouts of the Carolina

Coastal Pines. It covered basic dance steps, as well as practically applied creative components. Hundreds of Girls Scouts experienced the program, and it was fun to see their excitement and enthusiasm for it.

- I choreographed a flash mob for the Susan G. Komen Foundation. Hundreds of women and men of all ages and experiences came together, wearing pink, to perform this fun routine to "Shout!" by the Isley Brothers.

During our most intense, competitive years, I lost sight and focus on these types of experiences, which is unfortunate because they were so meaningful. Quality education shouldn't be reserved for hypercompetitive "winners"; instead, we should make the impact of dance and the performing arts available to as many people as possible. We need to return to the commonality of community.

In the past few years, we've reinstated our Girl Scouts and outreach programs and choreographed for a variety of fundraisers and groups. We are IN the community in as many ways as possible, spreading our love and passion for dance. While the localized experiences were great, I also wanted to keep our students abreast of the professional, working side of the entertainment industry.

Over the years, I acquired several friends and colleagues who are working in the entertainment industry and are willing to share their knowledge with our dancers. Building relationships is so important in building your business. It is amazing what people will share and do to positively perpetuate their expertise and craft.

Early in our competitive days, we brought guests to the studio to teach at our Intensives. They were amazing with exceptional credentials, but the series never gained the traction I wanted. When we were all in to the competition industry, we didn't have the time or resources to continue offering these experiences because our clients were spending so much money on dance competitions.

With a more fiscally responsible and manageable program, we created the opportunity for curated, experiential activities. We could bring high-level, professional-grade exposure and experience directly to our students in New York City. I aimed to create a dream experience for our Intensive Training Program students that was affordable, highly educational, intimate, and beyond anything that is offered via tour groups or the mainstream market.

Our experiences have ranged from classes with Broadway show performers and choreographers, to upper-level executive leadership training, to costume house tours and backstage/behind-the-scenes Broadway experiences. The classes are structured as they are at home—we rent space, we set the schedule, and approximately fifteen students are in each class. The cost is around the same as a competitive weekend, but the return on investment is priceless.

Currently, the trip is slated for every other year, but with its increasing popularity, it may become an annual event. Our families pay the studio for the workshop cost (which includes teaching fees and space rental), and we offer a la carte options (shows, tours, etc.). For the travel component, families decide how they'd like to travel (air, train, car) and determine where they'd like to stay (as travel preferences vary greatly). We schedule facilitated meet-up times while also making sure families have time to enjoy the city on their own.

Every time we plan the trip, we evaluate pieces that worked and ways it can improve. For example, the first time we did the trip, we attempted a group meal prior to a Broadway show. What a nightmare! It was complicated, took too long, and stressed people out. The following time, we eliminated group meals, and it worked much better.

At the end of each trip, I receive such immense gratitude from our families. One time, a mom looked at me and genuinely said, "I am so proud of you for doing this—you have changed our daughter's life." I had to hold back tears as I downplayed my response. The power of perseverance is in the payoff. Hang tight—you'll get there!

When an overwhelming wave of "rightness" washes over

you, it is so easy to push forward. Keep creating those experiences—small, grand, and everything in between. That's building community and commonality, and that's what people remember long after the dance is done.

## EMPOWERMENT

When we first initiated the transition out of the competitive market, one of our studio moms asked if I'd consider creating a leadership program for girls. I was flattered at the thought and wholeheartedly stood behind the idea. The timing didn't feel right, and I wasn't ready to dive in. I was too busy thinking about the performance, service, and experience piece to fully focus on the empowerment piece.

The idea was always very appealing, and it sat with me for a couple of years. Socially, the #MeToo Movement was heightening. I became hyperaware of our ability to offer action-oriented training that would provide training and skills for girls' success in anything they chose to do. We had a captive audience, and it felt right.

How could we place emphasis on training and skills to curate an action-oriented response for future generations? Let's learn from the past, so we can improve our future.

When thinking of names, I wanted to stay away from the notion that anything about girls needs to be helped or fixed.

Intrinsically, we are all capable of achievement, especially if we are supported, nurtured, and trained. Again, it was our opportunity to grab the idea and move the needle.

In the summer of 2018, when I was speaking at a conference in Arizona in front of hundreds of fellow dance educators, I decided to announce that I was launching a girls' empowerment program called Girls Geared For Greatness.

Manifest, and it will come.

On that day, I had no idea what the program would look like. The logistics were not hashed out beyond the fleeting thoughts of my brain. There's no better way to get the ball rolling than to throw it out into the world. When I left Arizona, I started looping in my friends who expressed an interest in helping with the initiative, and we got to work. Everyone was excited about the possibility because this naturally felt like the next step in our evolution.

In October 2018, we had our first Girls Geared For Greatness event. In our first year, we reached two hundred girls—dancers and nondancers—through our in-person programming, which included topics on leadership, perseverance, branding, and entrepreneurship. Successful women in our community donated their time to speak to our students about their unique journeys, successes, and challenges.

More surprising, people were calling from around the world inquiring about this program. For many, it seems like "one extra thing to do," but it is an extra thing with so much potential for purposeful impact.

With Girls Geared For Greatness initially sheltered under Stage Door Dance, we quickly realized we had something really unique, special, and popular in front of us. Girls Geared For Greatness applied for its independent nonprofit status and is looking forward to a future standing on its own two feet. Ah, so exciting! So unexpected!

Do you want to know one of the most exciting parts of this program? It brought girls back into our facility who left amid the competitive drama. They still choose to train elsewhere (or have opted out of dance completely), and that's okay. The damage was done in that part of our history, and my heart is at peace with it. To know the students (and their parents) are comfortable being in our building communing over girl empowerment and progress—that's a remarkable achievement. In fact, that is inner peace.

For the next phase, we are rolling out digital modules to connect with a wider audience of girls, colleagues, and networks in other cities, states, and countries. We will also offer in-person, executive functioning workshops, so we can continue pushing progress for the confidence, branding, and life skills of girls in our community.

We've also started the process of collaborating with local businesses and organizations and once the organization officially develops into its own entity, I cannot wait to see the level of impact it will have. The journey is just beginning, and I am excited to see where it will go.

In the next fifty years, I hope this program looks like a modern adaptation of the Girl Scouts.

## MYTH BUSTING

The top myth to debunk is the idea that you cannot train dancers at an exceptional level unless you participate in dance competitions.

Our students have been a part of the following since 2015:

- *The King and I* on Broadway
- The *Matilda* National Tour
- *A Bronx Tale* on Broadway
- *Harry Potter and the Cursed Child* on Broadway
- *The Ferryman* on Broadway
- The OM Still Growing Pre-Professional Company
- Regional and Community Shows
- Academic Accolades

When our student Will booked three Broadway shows back-to-back at eleven years old, his mom didn't talk about his competition scores or trophies. Instead, right before his Broadway debut, she called to thank me for the choreography that required him to remove his jacket midroutine. In that call, she also apologized for being so demanding about it. Now, he was in a show that performed eight times a week, and in his solo number, what did he have to do? He had to remove his jacket. She said, "You prepared him for that."

The affirmations continued as former students who moved to different states continue to lean on us for wisdom. Even better than that? Some students who left our programming eventually found their way back. The messaging that I'd known all along was reaching others, and it was slowly but steadily making its way full circle.

Many justify dance competitions as a necessary preparatory step toward working in the entertainment industry. The trophies don't prepare us for the reality of the entertainment industry; instead, they give us a false sense of accomplishment that isn't rooted in reality. In the entertainment industry, you must learn material at a moment's notice. You don't have months to polish and perfect routines for adjudication. You don't get to pick your best style. It requires the ability to conform to the overall vision of the creative team.

If you focus on excellence in training and opportunities in the above areas, the sky WILL be the limit. When you are making moves that are off the beaten path, there's no playbook detailing what comes next. It all goes back to the power of intentionally owning your narrative. Find an underlying statement that guides your professional and personal mission, and use it to the max. Big purpose has the power to lead to even bigger outcomes and impact.

Recognize your power and potential for change, and get excited about the prospect of the outcome. It won't be long until the wishes you initially envisioned are the actuality that's in front of you. Do not stop with the most obvious components of impact and change. Instead, dig deeper and delve into the dreams that didn't seem possible. Level up and exceed the expectations you set for yourself. Start small, dream big, and never stop working toward heightening your personal and professional standards.

# Chapter 8

# CHANGE THE GAME

When something could be better, ask: "What are you doing to fix it?" It is so easy to complain, vent, and feel frustrated without taking steps to improve the condition or circumstance. For the short term, it may feel easier to play the victim, but that's not a long-term solution for health, success, or happiness. What if every "gripe" that was posted on social media was exchanged for an action-oriented step toward positive betterment? Embrace a "change the game" mentality, and take the actions required. The work will speak for itself.

Somewhere along the way, I saw the following quote:

> "Confidence is quiet. Insecurity is loud."

Much like change, success also doesn't show up on your

doorstep wrapped in a package with a lovely bow. You pour your heart and soul into something, and guided reminders of your path gently nudge you in the right direction. When talking about journeys versus destinations, success is entirely a journey with hills, valleys, opportunities, obstacles, setbacks, and solutions.

I never wake up and say, "Wow, we did it! We got out of competition, and now life is so amazing!" Instead, my feet hit the floor and I hit the daily hustle as fast and hard as possible, working toward the goal and mission of creative innovation and impact through the performing arts. That level of vision and commitment is required to stay in the entrepreneurial game, and it is even more necessary if you are interested or focused on making pivots within your field. Complacency and stagnation are killers—avoid them at all costs!

In the past couple of years, there were a few interactions that signaled we were moving toward something exciting:

1.  My college scholarship program featured the studio as an entrepreneurial achievement. When I was sitting at the banquet table at their prestigious scholarship finalist interview weekend and saw the studio's logo, I nearly fell sideways out of my chair. In the day to day, it is hard to see the bigger picture, the greater impact. When others recognize it, it is thrillingly unexpected. In

that moment, every insecurity I ever felt about being an arts-oriented scholarship student disappeared.

2. A local business owner called our studio an industry disruptor. The comparative analysis: Stage Door Dance is to the dance industry what Airbnb is to the hotel industry. That's a pretty neat way to think of it. The changes I made weren't intended to disrupt; they were intended to improve my immediate piece of the pie. Yet, the movement has the potential to create waves, and that's exciting.

3. As I was doing an interview for the oral history archives of the state of North Carolina's "She Changed the World: Women Breaking Barriers" Project, the interviewer asked how it feels to be so successful at such a young age. I stumbled over the question because success is relative, and we still have so much work to do. The process is the progress, and I never take a single day of success for granted. I know that it can disappear as quickly as it appears.

4. I love being able to share our story with entrepreneurs and students, and I've recently been doing that a lot more. Out-of-the-box thinking and creative solutions have become my specialty, and I am grateful to share this knowledge with a variety of ages, businesses, and audiences. As I observe a world focusing on venture capitalism, I hope we never lose sight of the power of purpose-driven business.

These moments (and many others) represent what we have

accomplished, can accomplish, and will accomplish. I look at the day, month, and year, and question what's in front of us and how we can continue paving our way.

If you've made it this far in the book without throwing it in a corner and/or trashing my perspective on Dance Teacher Network or Competitive Dance Moms Chat, let's shift the conversation to YOUR power to create change.

You know the competitive dance industry has flaws.

If you are a studio owner or teacher, maybe you are interested in finding an alternative to competing for your studio. You recognize the dance competition industry is expensive, confusing, taxing on you and your families, and creates a lot of unnecessary negativity and stress. You're fearful of the consequences or gravity of navigating such a change, and yet, in your heart, you wish you could have more time and energy to invest in the overall success of your business. You might also like to prioritize personal time and family, which you are entitled and encouraged to do.

If you are a parent, maybe you are questioning your child's participation in dance competitions. You also recognize the expense, confusion, commitment, and stress, yet, you enjoy the social components and the validation it gives your child. At the end of the day, you want your child to learn, feel empowered, and gain confidence in their extracurricular activity. You trust your studio owner and instructor, and since an alternative hasn't been presented, you aren't currently aware of another option. If an alternative was available, you'd be open to considering it.

If you aren't a participant in dance education, maybe you have observed the competitive subsect as the forward-facing representation of the overall dance industry. Because alternative programs aren't often featured in media or news stories, you'd rather have your child involved in any extracurricular activity other than dance. I feel particularly passionate about dispelling this misconception.

These three populations exist because I've encountered them all:

1. The first time I told a large group about our competitive exit and branding shift, a woman from the West Coast requested to speak to me privately after the talk. She was very interested in navigating this process for her studio but was fearful of the consequence and losing clients. Tearful and honest, her conflict was real.

2. I've had parents leave, try other programs (competitive and noncompetitive), and still return to us because they believe in the culture we are cultivating and the technique we are providing.

3. I've sat at tables with incredibly successful businesspeople where they shied away when I mentioned my career

was in the dance studio industry. After digging deeper, their opinions were formed because of the projection produced via hypercompetitive dance studios.

Bottom line: As a collective, we must stop allowing a third-party vendor to dictate the perception of our industry. Every season the complaints on social media are rampant. Yet, the discontent is always swept under the rug as we proceed with the status quo.

If you are experiencing frustration, the bottom line is:

You cannot stand for one thing and enable another.

So, what does it mean to Trash the Trophies? I am not suggesting we need to end all forms of competition. At the very heart of it, life is a competition, and I want my students to thrive and succeed in anything they pursue. If we teach the hustle, the discipline, and the quest for excellence in our programming, a healthy, competitive spirit that is combined with humility and empathy will prevail. In order to facilitate this type of growth, we must make sure our programming choices support the healthy cognitive, emotional, and physical growth of our dancers.

When we encourage participation in competitive arenas, let's make it:

- In a way that promotes philanthropic impact
- In a way that improves our communities
- In a college interview
- In a Broadway audition
- In a job interview
- In recognition of sportsmanship or impact

When you show up to something, will it matter tomorrow, next year, or in ten years? The platinum trophies you received four times in one regional season for a contemporary solo will never go on a resume. The stakes simply are not high enough for the value placed on these "wins."

As we packed up my childhood bedroom, I had no desire to keep any of my former dance competition trophies. I've heard the same from many of my colleagues. In fact, when I talk to similarly aged peers, many agree that they loved their dance studio experience. There's a shocking commonality in the anxiety and disdain many experienced over the competitive component. This was decades ago, so imagine what it must feel like for our current students.

Yet, the emphasis on the trophy remains.

- Parents want their child to have the insignia.
- The prioritization of wins and placement is often parent/instructor motivated versus student motivated.
- The children just want to dance.

## EXAMPLE 1

One time, we were invited to participate in a mock competitive event that was being used as a training simulation for employees of the competition. The scores and results were fake, which we communicated with our studio families in advance. We thought the event would be fun and beneficial because it would give our routines another opportunity to be on stage at no cost to our families.

The mock experience turned out to be a very telling sociological experiment as we were still receiving complaints and questions from the parents about the fake accolades. It was a nightmare! Even when the competition didn't exist, people could not separate the preconceived notion of the environment from the actual experience.

## EXAMPLE 2

Several years ago, *The Dance Exec* received a Dance Web Award for Best Dance Blog. For that recognition, I received a generic "Dance Web Award" trophy in the mail. The trophy has a black base and a globe on top, and it is very sturdy. A year or two after receiving the award, I started receiving Facebook messages with requests for this trophy to be mailed to an ailing child. I've never been one to attach myself to material goods, so I told the mom I'd investigate sending it. When I went to mail it, the shipping was over $100. The situation felt a little weird, so I pushed it to the back burner.

A few weeks passed, and I started receiving threats over the whereabouts of this trophy. When I blocked the first person who was messaging, a second person started messaging me. I was so alarmed that I reached out to the Dance Web Awards, which is based out of Australia. It turns out this is a common problem they encounter.

There's something about the trophies and the process that brings out the animalistic side of participants. Think about it: do the trophies in your business's windows cultivate the culture you want, or do they inadvertently set an expectation for competition over collaboration? What do these labels accomplish?

The few recognitions we keep, ranging from *Business Journal* plaques to college degrees, are tucked away, out of sight. My email signature lists few labels, and when I list my title, it is generally out of need for professional reference versus bragging rights. I want to be viewed as an equal to others because that's where we can find commonality, connection, and the opportunity for collaboration.

Are we taking caution to use that level of cultural alignment throughout our business? Or do we knowingly (or unknowingly) tout our recognitions while also complaining about the competitive dance industry and its processes? Figure out where you stand and where you want to go. When you find your unique potential for change, you will tap into your opportunity to change the game and improve your piece of the ecosystem.

*Chapter 9*

# BE BOLD

*"Boldness has genius, power, and magic in it."*

—JOHANN WOLFGANG VON GOETHE

Reinvention is often unchartered territory, which is simultaneously exciting and terrifying. In order to change the game, bold leadership is a necessity. It's what makes people trust and want to join your movement.

*Bold Business* identifies the ten traits that characterize bold leaders:

- Taking risks
- Challenging the status quo
- Driven by results
- Showing confidence in others and themselves
- Empowering others to succeed

- Able to delegate
- Acting ethically and responsibly
- Championing change and diversity
- Leading by example and with humility
- Believing in changing society for the better[14]

We all have differing degrees of these traits within us. Maximize the use of your strengths, and foster the development of your weaknesses.

This core statement will keep you on track as you navigate your reinvention/culture shift:

> You can stay competitive in your training and purposeful pursuits while excluding the competitive experience.

Say that a few times over and believe it with your entire being. Keep nurturing great technique, and reconsider the possibility of the competitive experience. If the dollars that were funneled into the competitive dance industry were invested in technique, training, business, community, and unmatched experiences, the entire outlook and perception of the dance studio industry would shift. You have the power to be a part of that change!

Throughout the previous chapters, we've talked about how

---

14   John R. Miles, *Bold Business*, September 20, 2018, https://www.boldbusiness.com/human-achievement/bold-leadership-what-does-it-comprise/.

hard this type of change can be. If you are ready for reinvention, then steady accountability and action must be your top priorities. Put a plan in place (with deadlines) and make it happen! Sometimes, we can be our own worst enemies, so take caution if you find yourself falling into these "excuse traps" for avoiding action:

- I don't have time.
- I'm too old.
- It is going to be way too much work.
- That's not the way we've done/do it.
- I will risk failure.
- People won't think my studio is good.
- I'm known for my competitive program.
- People will judge me.

Guess what? People are judging you anyway. That's a reflection on them, not on you. As a bold leader, you are opening and inviting judgment because you are taking a stand for a cause you wholeheartedly support. Take pride in that, lean into your supporters, and be prepared for the challengers. Bold moves create discomfort.

Now, let's get going! Stop with the excuses, negative self-talk, complaints, and blame, and start taking control. You are the captain of your ship, and you deserve to reach the level of greatness you can achieve. When you are working toward your true passion and purpose in a bold way, it is going to feel great. It just takes a little bit of time and a lot of patience to get there.

# Chapter 10

# SHOW YOUR STRENGTH

Bold leadership is a lifestyle choice that requires strength, tenacity, and clarity. Being bold will rarely feel easy, as there will always be other challenges that arise. One big decision doesn't give you a "get out of conflict free" card. Life is full of varying shades of chaos and change. By activating this level of growth and development, you will feel empowered, prepared, and confident when other problematic scenarios enter your space. The solution to the problem will be easier to identify and address because you have a clear understanding of who you are, what you represent, and what you will tolerate.

While our overall studio culture improved significantly after our competitive industry exit, there have been other hurdles to navigate and address. The bright side? Our team is equipped and prepared to handle whatever comes our way. Powering through challenges builds loyalty and razor-sharp focus, and it starts with your leadership.

When handling conflict, use the following mantras as guiding principles:

- Be Proactive instead of Reactive: How can you get ahead of situations so you can control the narrative?
- Respond versus React: You control your intake of information. Make sure you are responding instead of reacting to maintain control over YOU.
- Focus Forward: Use the past as a reference point for lessons learned, but do not dwell on what is behind you. Keep your focus forward.

Everyone encounters challenges. The way you handle and move past them is what truly speaks to strength and leadership. When you're rocking the crazy days, know you are not alone and know that they will pass. Here are a few of our major post-competitive industry exit doozies:

### POWERLESS

Remember when I mentioned how much we love recitals at our studio? Imagine showing up at your recital venue for your tenth anniversary recital to discover that there was an electrical fire in the middle of the night, and your first two shows are pending cancellation because there's no power to the building.

The recital is THE huge capstone to the end of our year and the earmark of our program for hundreds of students. Our following season's enrollment is dependent on a successful weekend of shows. One misstep is detrimental to the entire business.

As I stood crying on the loading dock, other studios and performers entered their venues that are a part of the same complex. They looked at us pitifully. Several promised they'd be back to develop a collaborative solution. No one came back, so we took matters in our own hands and immediately went into action.

We were having our shows, power or no power. In the true spirit of the performing arts, we rallied together as a community, snaked electrical power out the back, and ran our first two shows off a generator at the side of the stage. We didn't have working lights, so we set up some Shakespearean-style footlights using the LED lights from the acorn that drops on New Year's Eve. You can't make this stuff up!

Stressed and sweaty, I walked on stage prior to each "powerless" show to explain the situation and share my gratitude and appreciation for everyone's support and understanding. At the end of the day, we celebrated our survival as well as the outpouring of goodwill. Nobody received a trophy. Instead, we received adaptability, resilience, community, collaboration, empathy, and discipline. We worked together, and we brought light into that building, in more ways than one.

On a day when we could have felt defeated and powerless, we left feeling more powerful and accomplished (and tired) than we have ever felt before. It was the most unimaginable, yet beautiful, example of our culture and community at work.

## THE BEAUTY OF BOUNDARIES

As your movement grows, you will likely have a minority percentage of your population challenge, question, or fall out of line with your programming requirements. That's okay, and it is to be expected. When you know what you represent, it is easy to identify a culture clash.

With boundaries, there does not have to be any ill will toward the conflict because the focus is on an amicable resolution for both parties. Avoidance never solves the problem, and communication is key in seeking resolution. It's not convenient or fun, but it is necessary.

Even though we are now noncompetitive, the competitive

attitude we discourage has made its way back into our space a handful of times. Specificity in all communication regarding your positioning is key in offsetting conflict. To gain respect, the positioning must be unwavering and fairly applied to all parties.

Questions are as varied as parental concerns about their child's positioning in a formation or routine to blatantly degrading feedback about our business operations. I always (try to) engage the parent in immediate conversation to determine their intent. I try to listen to understand versus listening to reply.

What's causing these feelings?

- Misunderstanding
- Miseducation
- Entitlement
- Misrepresentation
- Overcompensation
- External frustration

Once the root of the problem is identified, it is easier to approach the plan of action. Many times, conflict can be resolved with education and communication. Frustration tends to brew when there are unknowns.

In extreme circumstances, where it is impossible for the

business and the client to find a common ground and resolution, it may mean a parting of ways. As a businessperson, it is important to emphasize that I never want to lose a client. Ever! I also want to make sure that our clients are the right clients for our philosophy and culture. This creates a happier environment for all and is an important lesson I learned during our rebranding process.

While I try to be very pragmatic in my approach, that does not always mean the other side will be equally rational or understanding. People have accused me of being a passive aggressive, full of myself, bad at business, hypocritical bully. This is generally after they recommend an extreme solution for how they'd perfectly run my company (e.g., fire the entire team!), and I explain how and why that is not a solution.

Remember: when you stand for something, it will resonate differently with others depending on their experiences, circumstances, and projections. Their reaction is on them, not on you. Avoidance of problems is not the answer, and client solutions are not always the best solutions for the overall business. Clients are advocating for themselves. You have the duty of advocating for the bigger picture and the interest of all students, their family members, the staff, the brand, and the general needs of the organization. In order to do this effectively, boundaries are key.

## GETTING OUT OF YOUR WAY

As we entered year eleven in our dance studio business, my main goal was greater autonomy, empowered leadership, and strategic, efficient systems. This would be a necessity for us to scale and reach our target growth while also allowing me to develop vision and direction.

Because I am immensely curious about all things business, I took an industrial engineering workshop on LEAN systems because I enjoy studying the success, history, and stories of other companies, particularly companies that are nondance-related. Continuing education keeps us relevant, engaged, and open to new and creative solutions and implementations in any field.

At the end of the course, I asked the instructor:

"What is the number-one problem you see in productivity and efficiency for teams?"

His answer:

"The owner gets in the way of the company's success."

What a perfect affirmation for continuing my quest to empower others! If that class had been offered a few months earlier, I might have felt personally attacked. However, in working with a therapist and business coach, I already recognized I was hindering our studios' ability to scale because I kept infusing myself in the day-to-day tasks.

I've always believed that dance studios can operate as professionally as the most respected businesses. In fact, that was the premise of *The Dance Exec*, which offered free resources to elevate the industry. At one of my speaking engagements, two ladies approached me after a session to show me a notebook containing numerous articles they printed from *The Dance Exec* site. They said they used the resources to open their own studio and wondered who this crazy lady was posting all this info online and for free. My jaw nearly hit the ground. I was flabbergasted in the best way.

I had no idea anyone was applying the information on the site, and in that moment, I recognized the reach we can achieve. When *The Dance Exec* was at its peak, I was still very much in my own way. Self-awareness is a necessary component in growth, even when you're learning things about yourself that aren't super flattering. That's one of the reasons I stepped away—I had to get out of my own way.

Your windshield is bigger than your rear window for a reason. Learn what you can, when you can, and apply it to your bigger purpose. Then, share it. You never know when parts of your story (even the imperfect moments) will inspire and influence someone else.

## EXPERIENCE IS WISDOM

Ironically, on the day I started writing this chapter, I discovered an article in *The Wall Street Journal*. It said: "CEOs enter their golden years once they've accrued deep institutional knowledge and dealt with several s!@* storms—and that usually takes at least 11 years."[15]

Malcolm Gladwell corroborates this theory with his 10,000-hour rule, saying that to truly master a field one must practice the task for 10,000 hours, twenty hours a week for ten years.[16]

In a world that is saturated with self-help, self-care, earn tons of money, and love your life on the fast track mantras, look at the stories of the people who aren't in your face. They are the ones who are typically in the trenches, living the stories, wrestling and overcoming hardship, working super hard, and making a meaningful impact on the world.

Be wary of falling prey to the epidemic of hustle porn. Comparison is the thief of joy, and if you find yourself venturing down the rabbit hole of comparison, stop. Whether you are comparing your business, your talents, your child, or your perceived success or lack thereof, it's probably not healthy

---

15    Chip Cutter, "New Thinking Emerges on Optimal Tenure for a CEO," *The Wall Street Journal*, February 3, 2020, https://www.wsj.com/articles/new-thinking-emerges-on-optimal-tenure-for-a-ceo-11580725800.

16    Malcolm Gladwell, *Outliers: The Story of Success* (New York: Back Bay Books, 2011).

or productive. Take control over your behavior and your usage of time. Keep your eye on positive, productive action.

Remember, success:

takes time.

takes energy.

takes failure.

You will "fail" more than you succeed. But you will keep trying, and in the effort, you'll discover opportunity and victory that is far sweeter.

In the past year, I've received rejection letters for four supplemental job opportunities (including one where I was invited to apply) and have been declined for speaking opportunities via Ted Fellows (twice), TEDx, and Alt Summit. Managing rejection is an art, and putting yourself out there is what keeps you in the arena.

In that same year, I've presided over the creation of a non-profit, booked several speaking engagements, wrote a book, brought back *The Dance Exec* style work via TutuTix, and focused on my businesses. I've also identified ways to be more present in my personal life and more available to my tribe. That's a victory, too! And, yes, I also sleep, work out, and eat three meals a day. Time management is an art, and I'm lucky to have mastered it. A lot of that discipline comes directly from dance!

Our years and our victories/failures will look different. The only person we are competing against is ourselves. Our strength lies in the power to continue pushing forward. If you are always "winning," you need to find higher stakes. You have the strength, and now is the time to show it.

*Chapter 11*

# PAVE YOUR PATH

The world is very loud and demanding. You must find a way to position your vision and activate your messaging. Using words and actions to separate yourself from the noise, you can stand out in a society that begs you to fit in.

Personally, it feels good to be on the outside of the competitive dance industry. I can watch intense dialogue happen and feel removed because it isn't applicable to us. We are doing our own thing. I'm listening, but I'm not a part of it. I decided I didn't want to be a part of the noise and paved my own way.

While my heart aches for the potential of what the competitive dance industry could be, I also recognize the reality of its existence is not rooted in my vision for dance education. If negative perception of your brand is a possibility via affiliation with an external industry, you'd be remiss not to be strategic in considering your positioning. How do you align? Do your actions match your words?

In considering actions, words, and noise, take an inventory of how you spend your time and energy. With time being our most precious and valuable resource, you owe it to yourself to make sure you are spending it in the right places and with the right people. Information can be transmitted to mass audiences in seconds. It is important for your actions to align with your beliefs and brand.

Because of this "judge now, ask questions later" societal state, it is critical that we work to our fullest potential to promote our external storytelling. For our business, our clients, and our dancers to know who we are and what we represent, but it is also important to promote our mission to those who maybe didn't know our platform.

In changing your messaging, you must work extra hard to correct the assumptions people have already made and formed about your brand. We had to get to work on telling people about our exit from the competitive dance industry and the varying phases of the #BeMoreAtStageDoor existence.

Ways to spread your narrative include the following:

• Merchandise

- Testimonials and reviews
- Guest blogging
- Expos/events/fairs
- Story-driven email campaigns
- Curated social media
- Public speaking
- Magazine articles

In our studio's branding, you will never hear comparative language, such as "best dance studio." Opinions are relative. Do I believe we are the best dance studio? Of course, I do. I also recognize that we may not be the best option for every family.

This is the marketing blurb we currently use:

> Stage Door Dance Productions is reinventing the dance education model in Raleigh, NC. With a strong belief in age-appropriate instruction and choreography, the studio uses technique, performance, community, and character to encourage dancers to "Be More At Stage Door!"

Under the direction of Chasta Hamilton, the studio features two locations, in Brier Creek and at Lake Boone Trail, and six satellite programs as well as their unique Intensive Training Program and affiliated nonprofit, Girls Geared For Greatness. From a toddler's first recital to a student's first Tony Award, they are ready to dance alongside you every step of the way!

All facts. All concisely written and easy to understand. We change it regularly because our business is always changing. If you are standing still, you cannot reach your fullest potential.

Deep down, I believe the industry recognizes the need for change. The mumbling is there, and now, the action is required. Will the industry choose to make the shift? If so, what is the tipping point?

There's the very real possibility of a bubble burst. When a market becomes oversaturated, this threat is real. Remember when there were frozen yogurt shops on every corner, and then there were none? If you reference the list of dance competitions on DanceCompetitionHub, the number of competitions listed is fascinating and growing on a seasonal basis. With no prerequisites for market entry and no immediate overhead, the startup is relatively easy, and with consumer support, the cycle continues.

Despite competitive dance industry expansion and growth, the tension between studios and conventions/competitions is escalating. Recently, there have been more articles in dance media about sticking with your studio for training and being wary and mindful of overtraining in the competitive and convention market. In 2019, *Dance Spirit* magazine published an article titled "The Case for Staying with Studio Training." In the article, it mentions that weekend convention FOMO ("fear of missing out") is "spreading through studios like wildfire." Industry experts agree with the importance of prioritizing studio training, citing technique, physical safety, support system, staying power, and alternative options as reasons.[17]

While I opted out law school, I am frequently told that I can argue my way out of a paper bag. Nobody wants an external entity to negatively impact their business. The state of the competitive dance industry versus my business and brand was clearly so misaligned from my goals and my intentions in my business that I had to pave this undiscovered path.

When we made the choice to exit the competitive market, I wasn't thinking of any of the following catchphrases:

- Level up
- Scale
- Pivot
- Strategic vision

Now, these words have been used to highlight our story, our achievement, and they can be used to highlight your story, too. They're power business catchphrases, and while the process of paving a path can feel scary, it is possible.

---

17    Haley Hilton, "The Case for Staying with Studio Training.," *Dance Spirit Magazine*, June 20, 2019, https://www.dancespirit.com/the-case-for-staying-with-studio-training-2638932250.html.

When we decided to make the change, I wasn't looking for greatness. It was more for survival and purpose. I wasn't chasing the label of "game changer." I simply wanted to get back to doing what I love, and I wanted to be in full control of our trajectory and direction. When I reflect on the time immediately prior to our competitive industry exit, I feel sad and remorseful. I failed as a leader in the short term, but I discovered my strength in order to make it right for the long term. And I am stronger and more confident because of it.

Take your actions, your words, and the noise that keeps you up at night and determine how you will level up, scale, and pivot a strategic vision that fits your passion and your purpose. You'll pave a path, and you will make this world a better place.

# Chapter 12

# LET'S LAUNCH IT!

Right after I opened the studio, I had it in my head that one day I'd write a book called *Tutu Town* because I envisioned dance studios as the heartbeat of the modern American community. This book never made it to fruition and eventually became the foundational platform for *The Dance Exec*.

As I recently read the draft of *Tutu Town*, I found it to be naively optimistic. At that point in my career, I had nowhere near the experience required to write a book, and I'm glad the draft was abandoned and never finished. I'm grateful I can sneak a peek at my mind and thoughts in the early days because that hyped-up level of "unicorn crack optimism" has led to my success.

Within the sugar-coated optimism, I also noted this paragraph of real talk:

Words do not begin to capture the effort, sweat, stress, tears, anxiety, fears, and excitement felt throughout the process. In fact, there hasn't been a day since the studio was conceived that I have not felt that incredible spectrum of emotions. I have worked more than I thought was imaginable; I have dealt with situations I never saw possible; and, I constantly feel the pressure to work harder, be better, and progress and evolve in an industry that is constantly changing and developing.

These feelings are intense. They were there in year two, and they may be even more intense in year eleven. With each year, I am more protective of what I have created and the direction we are going. I do not want any outside influence to be a factor in our perceived value.

While *Tutu Town* may not exist, I wholeheartedly believe in the concept and power of dance studios as an empowering heartbeat of our communities. As you think about your positioning, which side of history you want your legacy to be on?

Most likely, you love performing and the process of giving or receiving dance education. In the right setting, the community it creates is unparalleled. If that's the case, take ownership of your circumstance and create an alternative to the competitive market. Remove the toxicity from your sphere, and carefully control how you are choosing to endorse your spending, in money and in time.

Your alternative option may not be identical to the alternative I created, but that's where creativity and innovation come into play. How can you adapt your program, training, and participation to best fulfill your purpose? If you are frustrated, exhausted, and upset with the havoc the competitive dance industry is wreaking on the success of yourself, your business, or your child, get out. Remember: complaints are not action.

Do you find yourself:

- Complaining or confused about adjudications/scoring?
- Stressed about feeling divided between different departments of your programming?
- Uncomfortable with the costume choices and intensity of routines?
- Exhausted by the travel schedule and expectations?
- Horrified about the financial expenses?
  - As a parent, how could you better spend that money?
  - As a studio owner, what if you could keep that revenue under your own roof? You'd have more funding for staff, programming, philanthropy, and business development. This would also directly impact your company's valuation.
- Concerned about the impact of the competitive environment on your students' well-being?
- Asking if there are better ways to elevate the heightened dance education experience and/or if a new activity may be better?

Then, what are you waiting for? Take control and head into action as a leader for your people.

Let's launch it!

1. Define your priorities.
2. List the ways you achieve those priorities.
3. Consider alternative methods.

Because I know you may still feel skeptical or uncertain or terrified (I did!), remember: most people do not want to spend ridiculous amounts of money to watch their child wear inappropriate costumes for hours on end on multiple weekends. In my experience, the parents seeking that type of environment are a terrible fit for our studio's culture, and they are in the minority. Even if you justify participation from the angle of "experience," that still doesn't work, because clients are spending hundreds (if not thousands) of dollars on these weekends. Experiences that can easily be duplicated and offer no immediate value or meaning cannot be justified at their current price point. It's a turnoff versus a sales point, and as you educate your clients, the new model becomes an easy sell.

I challenge you to step up as an innovator, dreamer, risk-taker, and game changer and fight for the things and visions you love. Because dance studios interact with an overwhelming amount of the youth population, we can redirect the future of society.

That's impact.

It is time we engage our creativity, enact change, and embrace ambition.

That's power.

Think your clients will lack buy-in?

I am lucky to have several clients who have stood by us for many years—in competition, in transition, and now on the other side. The Allen Family includes dancers Max, Hannah, and Avery. They moved to Raleigh in 2012 and have participated at the studio as students, in the competitive program, and in the Intensive Training Program. Their mom, Jamie, has inspired our culture development and growth in a variety of ways.

Her story:

"At age eleven, our oldest daughter participated in her first and only competition season with the studio. We hesitated for several years thinking that she wasn't old enough, that we couldn't afford it, and that our family didn't have time. By the time she joined the team, we had this sense she was already "behind." Most of the team began competing when they were six and seven years old. Some of them began competing as young as five years old. From the beginning, there was a mentality that this is the route we needed to take for our daughter to be a successful dancer. And maybe she would have a little fun doing it.

We had a fun year experiencing this side of dance, but I wondered, to what gain? My daughter experienced top-notch instruction while being surrounded by a few hundred other students. She got to compete with several ensembles on a variety of stages surrounded by lights. She loved the costumes and the opportunity to compete, but the criticism from the judges was so subjective that she hardly knew what skills she should work on for the future dances. Our studio didn't show as much skin nor dance as provocatively as other studios. The message communicated to our dancers wasn't about ability; it was about style or what everyone else was doing. Unfortunately, several parents jumped in on the negative bandwagon. They complained that our kids weren't winning enough and questioned all the decision-making from our studio instructors. At the end of the day, my daughter enjoyed being with her friends and dancing. We realized there are a lot of other ways to experience those same things without the negativity and subjective criticism.

As our studio took a shift out of the competition world, many of the dancers and parents grumbled and left the studio to find places to compete. We struggled with what the future would look like, but at the end of the day, we felt like our kids were valued and known; thus we decided to stay.

The shift for our family has been extremely rewarding. Where the competitive circuit becomes repetitive, our studio has the freedom to encourage students to engage in a variety of artistic endeavors. Two of my children have been involved in a professional musical theatre production because of community networking of the studio and director. They have taken multiple master classes from Broadway performers and choreographers with classes as small as eight to ten students at a time. We have traveled to Washington, DC, and New York City to participate in parades and musical theatre workshops and experiences. Instead of paying convention and competition fees, my kids are having tremendous life-filling experiences that instruct them in the present and will last forever.

They are also learning the importance of community engagement and how they can use their passion in the dramatic arts to empower the world around them for change. They participate in dance-a-thons and benefit shows to raise money and awareness to help change the world for the better. These kids are remarkable humans and given the opportunity, are making a mark in this community.

There are moments when our kids wonder if their friends are better dancers than they are because of competing every weekend. As parents, we try to evaluate if this direction will ultimately help our kids pursue lifelong dance. We keep coming back to the same answer: our kids are learning the love of dance, they are learning technique, they are learning to be good humans, and they are having fun. It's so good to know there is another option. Studio owners have to take the risk to foster these new possibilities."

Think your staff will lack buy-in?

Courtney joined our staff at the end of our competitive tenure. A freelance instructor originally from Canada, she's been with us since 2014 while also operating her own successful contemporary company, OM Grown Dancers. Since she's a freelance instructor, she frequents a variety of studios and scenarios. Anytime I feel curious about the scene, I go to her. In 2019, she told me she was stepping away from competitive studios after experiencing the following scenario:

> "I'll never forget getting a call last summer from a local competitive studio owner asking me if I'd come and teach a class for her advanced competitive team. She specifically said, "The kids are really stressed about their upcoming national competition and are exhausted/bored of running and cleaning their dances so much. A hard class, packed with deep stretching, advanced progressions, and a feel-good combination would be ideal!"...It was at that very moment that this validated my decision to leave the competitive dance scene. Since when was a class filled with the above requests a treat, reward, or uncommon regiment in a dancer's training? Since

when did "running/cleaning dances" replace the fundamental components in a dancer's young training life?"

Think your peers lack buy-in?

Melissa and I met through Carolina Dance Masters. She's sharp as a tack and never had a competitive program. In 2016, when I hardly even knew what our new format looked like, she said she loved the idea and wanted to apply something similar at her studio. I encouraged her to go for it! Last year, we ran into each other at the National Cherry Blossom Festival Parade Performance in Washington, DC. When we hugged, I could feel the positivity of our programs colliding.

"During the spring of 2016, I had the opportunity to attend a workshop hosted by Chasta where she discussed her Performance Company Program. As a noncompetitive studio, we had been looking for ways to provide additional performance opportunities for our students along with educational, service, and community-driven dance education. Chasta's program seemed like a great fit for us, and we began the MKSD Performance Company in the fall of 2016 for dancers who were dedicated to increasing their dance education and performance opportunities. Our studio used Chasta's program as a starting point and modified it to fit our individual needs, and it has been the best addition to our program since we opened over twenty years ago. Our students have danced at Walt Disney World Resort, Washington, DC, and been invited to dance at numerous festivals and charity events in our community and surrounding areas. We are currently planning our second trip to Orlando for another performance opportunity. The dancers have matured both in their technical skills as well as in civic understanding through charitable support we provide each year to an organization of their own choosing. Thank you, Chasta, for sharing your program with us—we couldn't be happier with its success!"

Even my friends who are heavily involved in the competitive industry encouraged me to make the move. That's a huge green light to GO! Whether you are competitive, noncompetitive, successful, struggling, itching to make some changes, burned out, or defeated, a slight change in attitude and purpose can shift your entire narrative.

## FIVE STEPS TO ACTION

Use the following five steps to set yourself up for success:

1. Keep Solid Technique + Explore the Artistry. A common misconception is that studios/dancers who do not compete do not value excellence. That's not true.
2. Find the Performance Opportunities.
   A. Practicing performance is making progress in your art.
   B. Cultivate experiences that enable students to learn and grow.

3. Drop the Devices.
   A. Avoid becoming so entrenched in the digital sphere that you neglect to recognize the power of what can happen within your life and your walls.
   B. Work instead of watch. Live instead of linger.
4. Infuse Essential and Executive Functioning Skills.
   A. Incorporate conversation about the multifaceted benefits of dance education.
   B. How can skills gained in the studio be applicable to everyday functioning?
5. Focus on the Teachable Moments.
   A. Achieve goals and celebrate. Miss goals and improve.
   B. Keep the conversation going about the power of the process.

Let's teach our students to be competitive, not on stage, but in life.

Encourage the use of their talents, energy, and critical thinking to change the world.

Inspire them to make an impact.

Let their skills from the dance studio enable them:

- To be cast in a show, but to continue auditioning and working hard when they are not

- To be confident in their college scholarship interviews and applications
- To be a leader within the studio and within their lives
- To challenge stereotypes when they don't feel right
- To acknowledge missed goals and use that as motivation for the future
- To master critical-thinking and problem-solving capabilities
- To maintain an incomparable discipline and self-awareness that will set them apart in every field and workforce
- To focus in a society with increased demands and shorter attention spans
- To develop healthy, meaningful relationships that last a lifetime
- To facilitate healthy, injury-free growth through exercise and proper nutrition
- To foster interpersonal relationships and skills over digital gratitude
- To universally gain understanding and empathy for varying mediums of performance

## LET OUR STORY INSPIRE YOUR STORY

When I think about my story and the studio's story, I'm grateful. Our story five years ago was a surface success story to the average observer. Yet, there was something deeper that had to be addressed. When the gut feeling hits, don't ignore it. Instead, dig in and do the work. Take OUR story and allow it to motivate and inspire YOUR story!

The work takes courage (and courage doesn't exist without fear), but igniting change is what keeps society moving forward. Change is the only constant in life, and if you embrace it instead of resisting it, the power is yours. While this change was about finding purpose-driven work beyond dance competitions, it brought so much more to the surface. Within the hardship and tears was the greatest gift I could have ever received: an unprecedented reinvention that captures everything I imagined as a child—a place where strangers become friends and friends become family.

Every card, every testament, every letter I receive in our new iteration is a treasure that captures the resilience of sticking with the journey.

It's the handwritten card from eight-year-old Sadie that says:

"Thank you for this studio, and for being the best teacher in the world."

It's the email I received from Nancy in 2018 that says:

"We have pulled together a solo costume for her...black jazz pants and I ordered a hot-pink sequin top which slightly shows her belly button at times when she dances...Caroline quickly informed me that, "Ms. Chasta expected her dancers to look 'classy' at all times and this would not be acceptable, Mom!"...We purchased a solid black bodysuit with clear straps to go under it so no skin shows no matter what!! Thank you for instilling that sense of decorum within her!!"

It's the holiday note I received from our graduating senior Rachel in 2019:

"Thank you for imparting the skills and mindset that have shaped my mind and career, not to mention life. Your influence has meant so much to me, and I can never thank you enough."

It's the texts from my colleague Amy:

"You can do nothing but go up and forward."

"It's in your genes."

"You were born that way."

It's the email from nine-year-old Victoria titled "Be More At Stage Door":

"A thought like this has to be proven, for everyone there should be movin and groovin. If this weren't true, then how can the place have a director like you?"

It's the mom who walked up to me on Recital Weekend and shared that their family is blessed to have found a studio appropriate to attend that does not conflict with their Muslim faith.

It's the cards that covered my office from floor to ceiling the day after my dog passed.

It's a tribe that bonded in the very best way through laughter, tears, tenacity, and patience.

Every staff member and family who supports our studio reminds me of our collective alignment in our mission to provide dance education that empowers, inspires, and changes the world.

What if our model became the standard versus the exception?

Let's use our movement to connect and create with others.

Let's expose people in positive ways to the power of dance.

Let's gravitate toward greatness.

Through our approach to education, let's highlight how this art helps us survive, thrive, and feel alive.

Kick out the dusty trophies.

Rev up your mission.

By turning pain into potential, I discovered one of the greatest opportunities in my life.

It soothed my soul, renewed my purpose, and awakened my passion. And I have a feeling it will do the same for you.

# EPILOGUE

Funnily enough, in one of the earliest draft versions of this manuscript, the book ended with something along the lines of "I wonder what my next opportunity for reinvention will be?" I deleted it and redid the ending prior to my first submission because it seemed so ridiculous. There was no way there'd be an opportunity for radical change presented anytime soon. At least, that's what I thought.

Spring 2020 was slated to be the most stacked, professionally fulfilling series of months I'd ever had. I was so hyped about it and the hard work required to get there. This was (finally) my time!

Then, on March 3, I started having a strange gut feeling about a trip I had scheduled to New York City. Covid-19/Coronavirus had recently made its way to the East Coast, and I couldn't silence this nagging feeling about the intensity we were about to face with this disease. On the morning of March 4, I decided I was being crazily overanalytical and would go despite my gut. After five flights were delayed for cancellations/being half-full, we threw in the towel and acknowledged it wasn't mean to be. (One day, I'll readily trust my gut.)

The days that followed rapidly intensified. A few weeks prior to realizing we would have to temporarily close our physical studio locations, I began thinking of alternatives for what we might do to keep our hundreds of dancers moving if we had to transition to a different way of instruction. It almost seemed silly to spend energy and time on a "doomsday game plan," but as a Type A overplanner, I explored many options. I'm glad I did.

On Saturday, March 14, hours before our local schools closed, we announced that we'd be transitioning to SDD Digital! We flipped the programming in forty-eight hours. There was no gap in instruction, and there was no stopping us. I was running 100 percent on adrenaline and lots of coffee. I was terrified and had to make a lot of quick leadership calls. I literally followed every step I discussed in this book, except I did it on a much faster timeline.

With the rapid, midmonth transition, it felt like I was starting my eleven-year-old business all over again. When I logged on to my first class on Tuesday, a Saint Patrick's Day themed Leprechaun Party, and I saw thirty-five, three-to-eight-year-olds ready to dance, I felt a calming sense of compassion that reminded me of WHY I opened my studios: COMMUNITY + CONNECTION. A total of 140 dancers moved with us on that Tuesday, and the numbers steadily increased each day that week.

Every concept and experience in this book allowed me to navigate this challenge as quickly and confidently as I possibly could. There's no playbook for how to respond to a global pandemic. Normalcy and routine are SO important for children during traumatic and upsetting times, and I was determined to create the most perfect platform for our students that complied with government regulations.

Of course, we had students leave the studios. Our satellite programs were all put on pause. I documented every drop, my heart aching as people were forced to make hard decisions due to job loss and other circumstances. Revenue went way down. Yet, in the hardship, I tried to keep an active, focus-forward stance to make sure we could guide ourselves through to the other side.

In moments of extreme panic and stress, we must center ourselves in an optimistic calm. We must discover what we know, even if it is in different, out-of-the-box forms, and we need to applaud those who are willing to journey with us as we navigate uncharted times. Because I felt so incredibly confident in our program and our mission, our transition was seamless and smooth. While we lost some students, we also brought in some new students to our programming. This new arm of the studio may even linger and evolve as a global piece of our studio. As unfortunate as the circumstances are and as stressful as the process has been, I am trying to view it as an opportunity versus an obstacle.

Throughout my experience, I was relieved I could focus solely on our programming and serving our students. We did not have to navigate canceled/rescheduled competitions, refunding fees, and parents upset over canceled competitions. This was a huge blessing in our ability to maintain a level of programming success within the pandemic.

The words of this book were written around our experience navigating away from the competitive dance industry. After navigating the pandemic, I realize there is so much power in this wisdom and advice that transcends dance competitions. The concepts presented apply to labels, awards, expectations, and social constructs that can collapse or be gone at a moment's notice. How do YOU guarantee your work is protected, preserved, and purposeful on a humanistic level? That's the ultimate question.

It is a question we will all consider more intensely as we

move into the future. From this situation, I can, without hesitation, proclaim that dance studios are fighters. We proved that we are one of the most creative, innovative, resourceful, and passionate industries in existence. In this situation, we flipped the switch and activated change at a moment's notice.

There's an Apple commercial titled "Creativity Goes On," and in the montage of snippets highlighting modified American life during the pandemic, there's a moment that showcases a digital dance class. The first time I saw it, it stopped me in my tracks. It made me think about the power of our staff, students, and families. Their adaptability, resilience, and willingness to keep dancing will be a memory I will forever carry with me.

Creativity goes on, my friends. It can outlast the competitive dance industry, our ability to be in our physical spaces, and the overwhelming fear and anxiety of the unknown. History will not forget how we reacted during this time, and I hope we use it as a catalyst to ignite more evolutionary, positive change in the future. Take that power and use it to impact the world. We can do hard things, and we can do them together.

# ACKNOWLEDGMENTS

Wow, it took a lot of people to get here. And, I mean A LOT. I am equally grateful and ransacked at the thought of trying to get everyone who has contributed to my success on paper. It simply isn't possible. You see, this book is a culmination of experiences, and people bring these pages to life. Thank you all for your role in shaping my story.

To JMM: My steady rock, thank you for teaching me the depths of love and the importance of setting boundaries amid the chaos. I love our life, and I love you.

To Aunt Cheryl: Within reason, there was never a "no" when it came to dance or going after my dreams. You dropped everything when I was nine years old to swoop in and maintain the most normal life I could have imagined considering the circumstances. You've always held me to the highest standards, and in return, you've always been steadfast in my corner.

To Granny: Your house was a haven for my creativity. Thank you for that safe space to thrive and your enthusiasm every time I'm on the stage.

To Elvis, Laila, and Scottie: Three dogs that have taught me more about myself and my ability to love than I could have possibly imagined in three very different phases of my life.

To the Scribe Tribe: You are some of the smartest people I know. You pushed me to be better, and I'm grateful. Thank you to my rockstar publishing manager Maggie (who is also a dance teacher!), Rachael for her incredible artistic vision, Zach for his marketing expertise, and the entire team for their contributions and support. I have learned so much from you.

To My Family—Wayne, Uncle Mike, Grandmother, Aunt Regina, Uncle Ned, Alex, Alexis, and Wanda: Having you all in the audience of my childhood shows, ranging from the living room to the dance recital, was always a treat. This story started with those simple shows.

To the Coombs (Jaimie, Brad, and Will): My second family. Dance brought us together and has gifted us the widest range of experiences possible. Life is so much easier with you all in my corner.

To My Staff—Sara, Amy, Brooke, Jana, Cheryl, Morgan, Haley, Courtney, Cindy, Annie, Brianne, Bryan, Guy, Christina, Emma, Hannah, Isabelle, Kayla, Maegan, and Rachael: I couldn't do any of this without you, and your support means more than I can express (especially this year—what a year it has been!). You deserve so much more than a "staff" label—you are allies, muses, challengers, and the steady pulse of this entire operation.

To Mike Cedar: My inspo buddy for over a decade. Thank you for always challenging me to do better and for always asking, "What's happening next?" and keeping me on my toes.

To Jack Barto: Before Stage Door Dance was even a thing, you were asking the tough questions. You've stood by through highs, lows, and everything in between.

To Stephanie Johnson, Elizabeth Ferguson, Sarah Whittenburg, Laura Page, Lindsay Shepherd, Liz Miller, Megan Booker, DJ Hardy, Kathryn West, Sandy Bridger, and Lauren Rainey: We may not see each other every day or every month or every year, but I love that we are always cheering each other on from afar.

To Nina Torano: Thank you for giving me the first opportunity for my own dance program those many years ago. We've been through so much together, and it makes me so happy that we are still going.

To Michelle: When you entered my life, I found the best studio buddy I could have imagined. Thank you for being my go-to for all things out of the ordinary.

To My Theatre Collaborators over the Years—Patrick Torres, Nikki Dyke, Ashlynn Hayes, Michael Santangelo, David Henderson, Ann Meigs, Thea Martin, Burgandy Trimmer, and Diane Petteway: Through our time in theatre, I have learned so much about the power of community. Thank you for that experience.

To Elizabeth Doran and the Team at NC Theatre: Being on your board of directors has been a lesson in great people working together to create exceptional strides and meaningful art. You inspire me.

To the Park Scholarship Staff of Past and Present—Laura Lunsford, Eva Feucht, Dana Dubis, Joy Tongsri, and Chaffee Viets: Your calculated perspectives on society encourage me to think brighter and broader.

To the Community at NC State, specifically Arts NC State, the Dance Program, and the Entrepreneurship Program: Thank you for sharing and supporting my story. I love being an alum of a community that fosters artistic, out-of-the-box thinking.

To My Dance Teachers—Joyce Daniels, Jamie Winter,

Brenda and Sandy Cicerello, Heather Brace, Kristy Pratt, and Debbie Corpening: You each instilled a fiery passion in my soul. You were authentic and nurturing and always pushed us to our greatest potential.

To My Teachers in TN—Teresa Byrd, Marilyn Dawson, Frances Register, Sue Solomon, Cindy Cobble, Yhona Jones, Brenda Winslow, Gail Franklin, Diana Thompson, Jan Bible, Barbara Morelock, Lloyd Morelock, Doug Lafollette, Susan Hankins, Phyllis Davis, and Mike Davenport: You all inspired my education, and I'm forever grateful for the many lessons you taught me and the opportunities you gave me.

To Jackrabbit and TutuTix: Thank you for being two amazing brands for dance studios. Our industry needs you!

To My Business Team—Jonathan, BP, Grant, Emily, Jess, and Areon: You all keep me on the straight and narrow and fill in all of the cracks where we need a little extra advice, support, or sparkle.

To the Allen Family: Thank you for so generously sharing your candid experiences and for being my Jiminy Cricket and sounding board over the years.

To the Junior League of Raleigh: Thank you for imparting so many additional training opportunities and skills that have made me the person I am today. You make such an impact on women in our community, including me. Richelle and Gail, I'm so grateful for your recommendation many years ago.

To the Women of City Ballet who nurtured me in my early career days—Sandy, Ann, Anne, Lisa, Julia, Janette, Suzi: I will forever be grateful for the lessons and guidance you provided.

To the Students, Families, and Alums: You all have made Stage Door Dance an amazing and magical place. Whether our paths crossed for one show, one year, a decade, or a lifetime, I treasure our time and memories together. Thank you for allowing me to be a part of your journey!

To the heartbreaks, the abrupt endings, and the relationships lost: I think about you occasionally, primarily with forgiveness and peace. You play an important part in this story, too.

Finally, there are a few people who left this world too soon; yet, the power of their memory pushes me forward: My mom (Karen), my dad (Russell), my grandfathers (Bill and Daniel), my special friend (Eugene), and my college advisor (Mr. Hall). Your lights are shining so bright from above.

# ABOUT THE AUTHOR

CHASTA HAMILTON is the owner/artistic director of Stage Door Dance Productions and the founder/president of the nonprofit Girls Geared For Greatness. She believes the performing arts can change the world, and she's on a mission to make it happen!

Recognitions include the Goodman Award for Regional Leadership Excellence in the Area of the Arts (2012), *Triangle Business Journal*'s 40 Under 40 (2014), Women In Business' Future Star (2016), and the Raleigh KNOW Tribe Featuree (2018 and 2019). In 2019, Chasta was recorded for the oral history archives for the state of North Carolina as a part of the "She Changed the World: Women Breaking Barriers" project.

She received her BA in 2007 as a Park Scholar at North Carolina State University. She currently lives in Raleigh, North Carolina, with her husband, John, and their Scottish Terrier, Elvis.

Printed in Great Britain
by Amazon

44872840R00138